Dr Penny Stanway p   a
child-health doctor before becoming increasingly fascinated by
researching and writing about a healthy diet and other natural
approaches to health and wellbeing. She is an accomplished
cook who very much enjoys being creative in the kitchen and
sharing food with others. Penny has written more than 20 books
on health, food, and the connections between the two. She lives
with her husband in a houseboat on the Thames and often
visits the south-west of Ireland. Her leisure pursuits include
painting, swimming and being with her family and friends.

By the same author:

The Miracle of Cider Vinegar
The Miracle of Lemons
The Miracle of Olive Oil
Healing Foods for Common Ailments
Good Food for Kids
Free Your Inner Artist

As co-author:
Breast is Best
The Lunchbox Book
Christmas – A Cook's Tour

Dedication

In memory of my mother, Joan Rench,
whose raised cakes and breads
were second to none.

THE MIRACLE OF
BICARBONATE OF SODA

Practical Tips for
HEALTH & HOME

DR PENNY STANWAY

WATKINS PUBLISHING

LONDON

This edition first published in the UK 2012 by
Watkins Publishing Ltd, Sixth Floor,
75 Wells Street, London W1T 3QH

A member of Osprey Group

3 5 7 9 10 8 6 4

Designed and typeset by Jerry Goldie Graphic Design

Printed and bound in Italy by L.E.G.O.

A CIP record for this book is available from the British Library

ISBN: 978-1-78028-106-3

www.watkinspublishing.co.uk

Contents

Acknowledgements

Thank you to my sister, Jenny Hare, for her joy in food and cooking; to my husband, Andrew, for his unstinting enthusiasm in discussing bicarbonate of soda and alkaline diets; to my family and friends for their good company and warm-heartedness when we eat together; to my agent, Doreen Montgomery, for her encouragement and support; and to my editor, Alison Bolus, for her patience, wisdom and common sense.

Introduction

Bicarbonate of soda (baking soda) is a white crystalline mineral powder with a multitude of uses, both domestic and commercial. It is also known as 'sodium bicarbonate', 'sodium hydrogen carbonate', 'bread soda' or, simply, 'bicarb'.

I have called it 'bicarbonate of soda' ('baking soda') in those chapters dealing with cooking, home hints and beauty, because this is the name most often used in these spheres of interest. However, in the rest of the book I have called it 'sodium bicarbonate', because this is how it is known by physiologists, nutritionists and doctors.

The names of certain other chemicals could sound confusingly similar to those unfamiliar with chemistry. These include:

- baking powder (which contains other ingredients besides sodium bicarbonate)

- sodium chloride (salt)

- washing soda (sodium carbonate or soda ash) and

- caustic soda (sodium hydroxide).

It is vital never to confuse any of these with sodium bicarbonate, so be sure that any container of white powder is clearly labelled.

Sodium bicarbonate is present (along with sodium carbonate) in the mineral known as natron, which is deposited from salt lakes in various countries. The ancient Egyptians used natron to clean their homes, their teeth and, when mixed with oil, their skin. They also used it to mummify dead bodies. Sodium bicarbonate can also be mined as deposits of nahcolite in rock, and it is present in the water flowing from many hot springs. Today, though, it is mostly produced in factories, mainly by a method that mixes salt (sodium chloride), ammonia, calcium carbonate and carbon dioxide in water. A total of over 1 million tons is produced this way each year in various countries, including the USA, Italy, Egypt and China.

Sodium bicarbonate is mildly alkaline in water but is also amphoteric, which means it can react with both acids and alkalis. It is useful in many commercial and domestic situations. It is used, for example, as a cake-raising agent, as well as to make baking powder, self-raising (self-rising) flour, soaps, domestic cleaning and deodorizing products, medications, water-softeners, 'dry' fire extinguishers and pesticides. It can also be used to make toothpaste and 'bath bombs' and to coat dental floss.

Last, but not least, our body's own internally produced sodium bicarbonate is a vital part of the acid–alkali balancing systems that keep us healthy. And by eating an alkali-producing diet and, perhaps, taking sodium bicarbonate or applying it to our skin, we can help to treat certain common ailments.

This important mineral is available in small quantities as 'bicarbonate of soda' ('baking soda') from supermarkets and grocery stores and as 'sodium bicarbonate' from pharmacies (drugstores). You can also buy it in bulk online.

CHAPTER 1

Household help

Bicarbonate of soda (baking soda) is a non-toxic product that can help to keep your home and laundry fresh, clean and fragrant. It can help in many ways and in many places around the home.

Cleaning products

Bicarbonate of soda (baking soda) is mildly abrasive and has degreasing, water-softening and deodorizing qualities. Keep it ready to use in a flour shaker. You can also use it to make the following cleaning products:

Basic Cleaning Fluid

Put 600ml//21fl oz/2½ cups warm water into a large bowl and stir in 1 tablespoon of bicarbonate of soda and two squeezes of washing-up liquid (dish detergent).

Use and storage: Make just enough for a particular cleaning job and use it from the bowl. Alternatively, pour it into a spray bottle, putting the top on only after any fizzing has stopped, and shake before each use.

Extra-strength Cleaning Fluid

To the Basic Cleaning Fluid recipe above, add either 120ml/4fl oz/½ cup white vinegar or the strained juice of two lemons. It will fizz a lot when first mixed.

Use and storage: Make just enough for a particular cleaning job and use it from the bowl. Alternatively, pour it into a labelled spray bottle, putting the top on only after any fizzing has stopped, and shake before each use.

It is unsuitable for waxed surfaces, or granite or other stone surfaces, because vinegar and lemon juice can cause dulling.

Basic Cleaning Paste

Put some bicarbonate of soda into a bowl and stir in enough water to make a paste. The amounts required depend on the size of the job. The proportions are about three parts bicarbonate of soda to one part water. Mix in a few drops of lemon, tea-tree, lavender or other essential oil for fragrance, if wanted. This is excellent for cleaning areas of adherent grime, such as a ring around a bathtub.

Use and storage: Make just enough for a particular cleaning job and use it from the bowl. If the paste starts to dry, add more water.

Extra-Strength Cleaning Paste

Make the Basic Cleaning Paste recipe above, but using vinegar instead of water.

Use and storage: Make just enough for a particular cleaning job and use it from the bowl. If the paste starts to dry, add more water.

Cream Cleaner

Make the Basic Cleaning Paste recipe above, then stir in extra water until it has the consistency of thick cream. Add a few drops of lemon, tea-tree, lavender or other essential oil for fragrance, if wanted.

Use and storage: Make enough for a particular job and use it from the bowl. Alternatively, pour it into a labelled squeezy bottle, putting the top on only after any fizzing has stopped, and shake before each use.

Scouring Powder

This recipe includes borax substitute (sodium sesquicarbonate), which is available online (for suppliers in the UK, for example, see page 129), and salt. The borax substitute has bleaching, stain-removing, deodorizing and disinfecting qualities, whilst the salt has de-greasing and cleaning qualities. Mix equal amounts of bicarbonate of soda, borax substitute and table salt in a bowl. Apply with a scrubbing brush, a cloth or, for small hard-to-reach areas, an old toothbrush.

Use and storage: Make enough for a particular job and use it from the bowl. Alternatively, put it into a labelled jar or plastic container.

CAUTION: if you're unsure whether a cleaning product will be safe on a particular surface, try it on a small, inconspicuous area first.

How to clean ...

Hands

Wash very soiled hands with soap, then sprinkle with bicarbonate of soda (baking soda). Rub your hands together, then rinse and dry.

Sprinkle bicarbonate of soda into rubber gloves to keep them fresh and make them easy to put on.

Sponges and cloths

Clean and deodorize sponges and cloths by soaking them in Basic Cleaning Fluid (above), then rinsing and drying.

Walls, doors, work surfaces, floors and furniture

Bicarbonate of soda helps to clean paint, laminate, other plastic, glass, granite, other stone, composite, rubber, brick, steel, fibreglass and washable wallpaper. If using it on bare wood, be sparing with the water and dry well to avoid water marks.

- Mop or wipe floors with 100g/3½oz/½ cup bicarbonate of soda dissolved in a bucket of hot water.

- Wipe other surfaces with Basic Cleaning Fluid (above), then rinse.

- Rub particularly soiled or stained areas with bicarbonate of soda on a damp sponge or cloth, then rinse.

- Banish grease or scuff marks on washable walls with bicarbonate of soda on a damp sponge; rinse, then wipe dry.

Dirty dishes

- Add 50g/1¾oz/¼ cup of bicarbonate of soda and the juice of ½ a lemon to washing-up water to aid de-greasing and help loosen stuck-on food. You'll need less washing-up liquid (dish detergent) than usual.

- Store steel-wool pan scourers in bicarbonate of soda to prevent rust.

- Clean the kitchen sink with Extra-Strength Cleaning Fluid (see page 2) or rub all over with bicarbonate of soda sprinkled on a damp sponge or cloth.

Sink pipes

- Help clear a block by pouring 200g/7oz/1 cup bicarbonate of soda down the plughole, followed by 240ml/8fl oz/1 cup hot vinegar. Wait for 30 minutes, then flush with a kettle of just-boiled water. If necessary, use a sink plunger.

- Freshen waste pipes and prevent them from becoming blocked by pouring 100g/3½oz/½ cup of bicarbonate of soda down the plughole and flushing with a kettle of just-boiled water each month.

Dishwashers

- Mix 2 tablespoons of bicarbonate of soda with 2 tablespoons borax substitute (see page 3) to make dishwashing powder.

- Help prevent unwanted odours by filling the dishwasher-powder (or tablet) dispenser with bicarbonate of soda and running a rinse cycle.

- Alternatively, clean inside and out with Basic Cleaning Fluid or Extra-Strength Cleaning Fluid and wipe clean.

- Or simply sprinkle 100g/3½oz/½ cup bicarbonate of soda into the bottom of the dishwasher after emptying it.

Refrigerators and freezers

- Clean a refrigerator or freezer by wiping inside and out with Basic Cleaning Fluid (see page 1), then rinsing. The remaining film keeps it smelling sweet.

- Rub stained areas with Basic Cleaning Paste (see page 2), then rinse.

- Make a refrigerator or freezer smell sweet with a bowl of bicarbonate of soda inside. Stir it every few days and replace every 2–3 months.

Wooden chopping boards

- Spring-clean a board by sprinkling it with bicarbonate of soda, then spraying it with white vinegar. Leave the bicarbonate-vinegar paste on for 30 minutes before rinsing with hot water.

- Deodorize a cutting board or wooden work surface that smells of garlic or onions by sprinkling some bicarbonate of soda on to a damp sponge, rubbing this over the board, then rinsing it clean.

Saucepans

CAUTION: Do not use bicarbonate of soda on nonstick pans, as it can damage the surface.

Get rid of burnt-on food residues by:

- brushing or scrubbing a saucepan with bicarbonate of soda or Scouring Powder (see page 3). Don't scour saucepans that have an enamelled interior.

- wetting the saucepan with hot water then sprinkling on a thick layer of bicarbonate of soda. Leave overnight, then brush or scrape off the residues.

- putting 240ml/8fl oz/1 cup water into the saucepan, adding 1 tablespoon white vinegar and bringing to the boil. Add 2 tablespoons bicarbonate of soda and wait for the fizzing to subside, then brush or scrape off the residues.

Oven and hob

CAUTION: The Basic Cleaning Paste can mark shiny stainless steel, and bicarbonate of soda can darken aluminium or corrode the heating elements in an electric oven.

- Spray the oven walls with water, then spread them with a thick layer of Basic Cleaning Paste (see page 2). Leave this on for several hours, spraying every hour or so to keep the paste moist. Use a spatula, palette knife or hob scraper to remove the debris. Wipe clean.

- Deal with charred greasy food residues on an oven floor by spraying with water, sprinkling on a thick layer of bicarbonate of soda and spraying again. Leave for several hours, spraying every hour or so to keep the paste moist. Wipe clean.

- If necessary, clean an oven or hob with Extra-Strength Cleaning Paste (see page 2).

- Clean a greasy hob, grill or splash-back by rubbing on bicarbonate of soda with a damp sponge or cloth, then wiping clean.

- De-grease and clean an encrusted barbecue grill by applying Extra-Strength Cleaning Paste (see page 2), leaving for several hours, brushing with a wire brush, then wiping clean.

Microwave oven

- Clean inside a microwave oven by wiping with Basic Cleaning Fluid (see page 1).

- Alternatively, put 1 tablespoon of bicarbonate of soda and 240ml/8fl oz/1 cup water into a microwaveable bowl and put this in the oven. Set the oven so the liquid boils for 3–4 minutes. Wipe the inside of the oven with a damp cloth or kitchen paper.

Bathroom

- When you have a bath, add 2 tablespoons of bicarbonate of soda to the water. This will help to prevent a scummy ring forming around the bathtub when you drain away the water.

- Clean the bathtub, basin, taps, tiles and mirrors by using a damp cloth or sponge to apply fragranced Cream Cleaner or Basic Cleaning Paste (see pages 2 and 3). Rinse.

- Alternatively, rub with bicarbonate of soda sprinkled on to a damp cloth or sponge, then rinse.

- For heavier soiling or to clean glass shower screens, rub on Extra-Strength Cleaning Paste (see page 2), leave for 30 minutes, then rinse. Dry a glass shower screen with a barely damp towel.

- Help prevent mineral salts in hard water blocking a shower-head by pouring 50g/1¾oz/¼ cup bicarbonate of soda and 240ml/8fl oz/1 cup white vinegar into a strong, hole-free plastic bag. Tie this around the shower-head and leave for 30 minutes. Remove, then run the water for a few seconds. (If you can remove the shower-head, simply immerse it in the above mixture for 30 minutes, then rinse.)

- Clean a lavatory cistern and bowl by putting 200g/7oz/1 cup bicarbonate of soda into the cistern overnight, then flushing next morning. Repeat once a month.

- Clean a lavatory bowl by sprinkling bicarbonate of soda on to a damp scrubbing brush and scrubbing under the rim.

- Treat a stained lavatory bowl by rubbing with Extra-Strength Cleaning Paste (see page 2).

- Use an old firm-bristled toothbrush to apply Extra-Strength Cleaning Paste (see page 2) to soiled tile grouting. Leave for 30 minutes, then rinse.

- For particularly grimy grouting, mix three parts bicarbonate of soda with one part bleach and scrub this over the grouting with a toothbrush. Wait for 30 minutes, then rinse.

- Clean a soiled or mildewed machine-washable shower curtain by putting it in the washing machine along with a large bath towel. Add 200g/7oz/1 cup bicarbonate of soda to the washing powder or liquid detergent. Then wash on a low-temperature setting, adding 120ml/4fl oz/½ cup of white vinegar to the fabric-softener dispenser during the rinse cycle. Don't spin fast, or the curtain could become permanently creased. Hang up to dry.

- Clean a non-machine-washable shower curtain by soaking it for 30 minutes in a bath of warm water containing about 150g/5½oz/¾ cup bicarbonate of soda. Rinse and drip-dry.

Baby and child equipment and toys

- Dip children's dirty washable toys into Basic Cleaning Fluid (see page 1), or use a cloth to wipe them with this. Rinse and dry.

- Wash a plastic paddling pool and remove any mildew with Basic Cleaning Fluid (see page 1).

- Clean high-chairs, car-seats, buggies (strollers) and plastic mattress protectors by sprinkling bicarbonate of soda on to a damp sponge, rubbing with this, then wiping with a clean sponge several times.

- Remove milk residues from a baby's bottles, teats (nipples) and bottle brushes by soaking them in Basic Cleaning Fluid (see page 1). Rinse, then sterilize as usual.

Fruits and vegetables

Many people wash fruits and vegetables before eating them to get rid of dirt, pesticide traces and micro-organisms. You could just use water, but a bicarbonate of soda solution is better.

- Wash fruits and vegetables in a solution of 1 teaspoon bicarbonate of soda dissolved in a bowl of water, then rinse.

- Shake a little bicarbonate of soda on to a wet vegetable brush and gently scrub firm fruits and vegetables.

- Clean soft fruits with a damp sponge sprinkled with bicarbonate of soda.

Metal

Bicarbonate of soda can help to clean silver, chrome and copper. It has even been used to clean the copper Statue of Liberty in New York.

Do not, however, use it on aluminium, as it would remove the thin protective coating of aluminium oxide. Bare aluminium reacts to acid so would soon look patchy if touched with sweaty hands or exposed to city air.

- Scrub a silver item with an old toothbrush and some Basic Cleaning Paste (see page 2). Rinse with warm water, dry with kitchen paper, then polish with a soft cloth.

- Put tarnished silver on aluminium foil in a bowl of warm water containing 1 teaspoon of bicarbonate of soda. (Or put the silver item into warm water in an aluminium container). Wait 5–15 minutes, then remove, rinse, dry with kitchen paper and polish with a soft cloth. Silver reacts with oxygen and sulphur gases in the air to form a tarnish containing silver sulphide. In turn, aluminium reacts with silver sulphide to form aluminium sulphide, leaving sparkly bright pure silver.

- Clean chrome on car bumpers (fenders) and hubcaps, or on a bicycle, by rubbing bicarbonate of soda over them with a damp sponge. Rinse, then polish with a soft dry cloth.

- Make stainless steel shine by rubbing on bicarbonate of soda with a damp sponge, then rinsing and drying.

- Clean brass or copper objects by rubbing with bicarbonate of soda sprinkled on to half a lemon. Rinse and dry.

- De-grime gold jewellery by putting it into a bowl, sprinkling it with bicarbonate of soda, then pouring white vinegar over it. Rinse and dry. However, don't do this if the jewellery contains pearls or if gemstones have been glued in place rather than captured in metal 'claws'.

Stain removing

For stains on clothing, see 'Laundering' (page 13).

Get rid of tannin stains from tea and coffee by:

- using a damp sponge to rub bicarbonate of soda (baking soda) on to cups and mugs, leaving for 30 minutes, then rinsing.

- filling cups and mugs with warm water and adding ½ teaspoon of bicarbonate of soda. Leave for 30 minutes, then rinse.

- filling a coffee pot or teapot with hot water and adding 2 teaspoons of bicarbonate of soda and 2 teaspoons of white vinegar. Leave for 30 minutes, then rinse.

- filling a glass and metal (but not aluminium) cafetière with hot water, stirring in 1 teaspoon of bicarbonate of soda and 1 teaspoon of white vinegar, and leaving it to soak for 30 minutes before rinsing.

- Clean fruit drink or fruit juice stains from kitchen work surfaces or other washable surfaces by spraying them with water, then sprinkling them with bicarbonate of soda. Leave for 30 minutes, then wipe clean.

- Remove crayon marks on a painted or papered wall by sprinkling bicarbonate of soda on to a damp sponge, rubbing the wall very gently, then wiping clean.

- Eradicate water spots on wooden floors by dabbing with a sponge or cloth dampened with Basic Cleaning Fluid (see page 1). Wipe clean and repeat several times to remove all traces of bicarbonate of soda. Dry well. Don't wet the wood too much, as this could simply make more water spots!

- Deal with a stained laminate (or other plastic) or marble worktop or other surface by rubbing on some Basic Cleaning Paste (see page 2), then rinsing.

- Clean a stained vacuum flask or one that you haven't used for some time by putting 1–2 teaspoons of bicarbonate of soda into the flask and filling it with hot water. Leave for 30 minutes, then rinse well.

- Remove wine, grease and certain other stains from carpet by lightly wetting the stains, then sprinkling them with bicarbonate of soda. Leave to dry, then vacuum up the residue.

- Apply Extra-Strength Cleaning Paste (see page 3) to ink stains on hard floors, then rinse and dry.

- Clean brown staining on the base of your iron by unplugging and cooling it first, then rubbing with Basic Cleaning Paste.

Laundering

- Keep your laundry basket fresh by sprinkling a little bicarbonate of soda into it each day.

- Clean your washing machine drum, and inside the door, with Basic Cleaning Fluid or, for stubborn marks, Basic Cleaning Paste (see pages 1 and 2).

- Deodorize your washing machine drum, and inside the door, by wiping with Basic Cleaning Fluid (see page 1).

- Alternatively, clean the washing machine by putting 50g/1¾oz/

¼ cup of bicarbonate of soda into the washing-powder dispenser and 240ml/8fl oz/¼ cup of white vinegar into the fabric-softener dispenser before running the machine on a short cycle.

- Add 100g/3½oz/½ cup of bicarbonate of soda along with your usual amount of liquid washing detergent to the washing machine or hand-wash bowl for more effective washing power. This also helps shift many sorts of stain.

- Home-make a fabric softener (conditioner) by putting 200g/7oz/1 cup bicarbonate of soda, 240ml/8fl oz/1 cup vinegar and 480ml/16fl oz/2 cups of water into a bottle large enough to accommodate the effervescence produced when bicarbonate of soda mixes with vinegar. Add 60ml/2fl oz/¼ cup of this mixture to your washing machine's fabric-softener dispenser when you do a wash, or put it into the final rinse water if handwashing. Bicarbonate of soda helps to make towels soft and fluffy.

- For a fragranced fabric softener, use the above recipe but add 3–4 drops of lemon, lavender or rose essential oil.

- Help to whiten white clothes by adding 100g/3½oz/½ cup of bicarbonate of soda to the washing-powder dispenser, or, if washing by hand, to the final rinse water.

- Alternatively, add 50g/1¾oz/¼ cup of bicarbonate of soda to a basin of cold water, immerse the clothing and soak overnight. Next morning, wash as usual.

- For greater whitening action, add the juice of a lemon and 50g/1¾oz/¼ cup of bicarbonate of soda to a basin of cold water. Soak the clothing overnight and wash it next morning.

- Alternatively, boost the performance of bleach by adding 100g/3½oz/½ cup of bicarbonate of soda and 240ml/4fl oz/½ cup of bleach to a bowl of water.

- Whiten cloth nappies (diapers) by adding 100g/3½oz/½ cup of bicarbonate of soda to the washing-powder dispenser, or along with the washing powder if hand-washing.

- Use bicarbonate of soda to make chlorine bleach more effective: add 100g/3½oz/½ cup along with the usual amount of bleach.

- Deodorize soiled cloth nappies (diapers) by putting 50g/1¾oz/ ¼ cup of bicarbonate of soda into a bucket of cold water and soaking them overnight. Next morning, wash as usual.

- If clothing is stained with something acidic (such as fruit juice or tomato sauce), pre-treating it with bicarbonate of soda before washing should prevent the acid eating into the fabric; it should also loosen the stain. Sprinkle with bicarbonate of soda, spray with water then leave for 30 minutes before washing. This is also effective for acidic sweat, vomit and urine stains.

- Remove a blood stain by putting 100g/3½oz/½ cup of bicarbonate of soda and 120ml/4fl oz/½ cup of white vinegar into a bowl of cold water and soaking the item in this mixture overnight. Wash as normal next day.

- Get rid of grease on clothing by applying a paste of bicarbonate of soda and water, leaving for 30 minutes then adding 100g/3½oz/½ cup of bicarbonate of soda to the washing machine (or a bowl if hand-washing) along with the liquid detergent. Run your usual cycle.

- Or make a paste from two parts of bicarbonate of soda, one part of cream of tartar and a little water and rub this on a grease mark before washing.

- Rub a tar stain with Basic Cleaning Paste (see page 2) then wash it with bicarbonate of soda and water.

- Remove a rust stain from clothing by soaking it in lemon juice then sprinkling with a thick layer of bicarbonate of soda. Leave overnight, then rinse and wash.

- Try eliminating a mildew smell from fabric by soaking it in Basic Cleaning Fluid (see page 1) overnight, then washing.

Deodorizing

Bicarbonate of soda neutralizes unpleasant smells. It acts against odours from acidic substances (such as in sweat, urine or vomit) and alkaline ones (such as ammonia from wet nappies/diapers).

For refrigerators and freezers, see page 6. For dishwashers, see page 5. For wooden chopping boards, see page 6. For kitchen-sink pipes, see page 5. For laundry, see page 13.

- Prevent unpleasant smells in a larder or store cupboard by keeping a small open bowl of bicarbonate of soda in it. Stir every few days and replace every 2–3 months.

- Eliminate stale smells from plastic bowls or food containers by filling them with hot water and stirring in 1 tablespoon of bicarbonate of soda. Soak for 30 minutes, then rinse.

- If the smell persists, repeat, adding 1 tablespoon of vinegar and a few drops of washing-up liquid (dish detergent) along with the bicarbonate of soda.

- Add a small handful of bicarbonate of soda to keep a kitchen-rubbish (garbage) container smelling sweet.

- Prevent unpleasant smells from your waste-disposal unit (garbage-disposer) by each week pouring 2 tablespoons of bicarbonate of soda and 1 tablespoon of white vinegar into it and running hot water from the tap as you operate the disposer.

- Make a stored blanket smell sweeter by shaking bicarbonate of soda over it, then rolling it up. Leave overnight, then shake it next morning and tumble it in the tumble drier set to cold.

- Deodorize carpets and rugs by shaking bicarbonate of soda all over them, waiting at least 30 minutes, then vacuuming.

- After cleaning spilt drink or food from a carpet, sprinkle with bicarbonate of soda, wait 30 minutes, then vacuum. This makes an unpleasant smell less likely to linger.

- Deodorize the carpet in your car by sprinkling it with bicarbonate of soda, leaving for at least 30 minutes, then vacuuming.

- Leave a small pot of bicarbonate of soda in each room to act as an air freshener by neutralizing any unwanted odour. Commercial air fresheners mostly act by producing a masking scent.

- Home-make a fragranced air freshener by adding a few drops of lemon, geranium, lavender, neroli, rose or other essential oil to a small pot of bicarbonate of soda.

- Neutralize a sour odour from cleaned-up human or pet vomit stains by sprinkling generously with bicarbonate of soda. Leave for several hours, then vacuum.

- Sprinkle bicarbonate of soda into smelly shoes, boots or trainers, leave overnight and then, next morning, tap out the surplus. (Note that doing this with leather shoes could stiffen the leather.)

- Keep a wardrobe (closet) smelling sweet by putting an open bowl of bicarbonate of soda inside. Add a few drops of lemon, geranium, lavender, neroli, rose or other essential oil for special fragrance.

- Alternatively, use scraps of fabric to make little bags which you can fill with bicarbonate of soda and, perhaps, some fragrant essential oil, tie up with string or ribbon, and keep inside a wardrobe or drawer.

- Sprinkle bicarbonate of soda into garment storage bags to prevent musty smells.

- Freshen stuffed toys by sprinkling with bicarbonate of soda. Wait for 30 minutes, then brush off.

- If there's a smoker in your home, put bicarbonate of soda into the ashtrays to combat the tobacco smell.

- Sprinkle tents, waterproofs and other camping gear with bicarbonate of soda before storing.

- Rid a vacuum flask of stale smells by filling it with hot water and adding 2 teaspoons of bicarbonate of soda. Soak for 30 minutes, then rinse.

- Help prevent odour from a pet's litter tray by putting a thick layer of bicarbonate of soda on the bottom of the tray before adding the litter.

- Also, sprinkle bicarbonate of soda over a cat litter tray to help neutralize unpleasant smells.

- To remove the wet-dog smell from a damp dog's coat, sprinkle with bicarbonate of soda, wait 30 minutes, then brush it out.

- Make a dog's or cat's bedding smell better by sprinkling it with bicarbonate of soda, leaving it for 1 hour, then vacuuming.

Rust removing

Help remove rust from metal by applying Basic Cleaning Paste (see page 2) with a damp cloth. Scrub lightly with a piece of aluminium foil, rinse and dry with kitchen paper.

Other

- If you don't have a fire extinguisher or a fire blanket at the ready, but you do have a large amount of bicarbonate of soda to hand, put out a small grease or oil fire, or an electrical fire, by throwing bicarbonate of soda over it. (Water is unsafe for either sort of fire). But don't use bicarbonate of soda on a deep-fat-fryer fire, as it could make the flaming grease splatter. Also, take no risks and, if necessary, get yourself and others out of the house and make sure that someone calls the fire service.

- Sprinkle bicarbonate of soda on to floors or worktops or in cupboards to repel unwanted insects.

- Remove smears left after cleaning dead insects from a car windscreen (windshield) by applying bicarbonate of soda on a damp sponge, then rinsing and wiping clean.

- Clean hairbrushes, combs, toothbrushes and make-up applicators by soaking them in Basic Cleaning Fluid (see page 1) for 30 minutes, then rinsing well.

- Spray plant foliage affected by mildew fungi with Basic Cleaning Fluid (see page 1) in the evening.

- To treat plant foliage affected by black-spot fungi, add 1 teaspoon of cooking oil to a bottle of Basic Cleaning Fluid (see page 1) and spray in the evening.

- Clean vases inside by filling with hot water and adding 2 tablespoons of bicarbonate of soda. Leave for 1 hour, then rinse.

CHAPTER 2

Cooking with bicarbonate of soda

Bicarbonate of soda (also called baking soda, bread soda or cooking soda) is a godsend for a cook. One reason for this is that when combined with water and acid, it creates tiny carbon-dioxide bubbles that aerate (raise or leaven) dough, batter or cake mix, making it puffier and lighter. Yeast and eggs were the main raising agents until the late 1700s, when scientists found that bicarbonate of soda acted faster. Bicarbonate of soda can be used:

- on its own, if the recipe contains an acidic food (see page 22) or cream of tartar (a powder that produces acid when mixed with water)

- in baking powder

- in self-raising (self-rising) flour.

Acidic foods that enable raising by bicarbonate of soda:

- Baking powder

- Beer

- Buttermilk

- Cider (apple cider)

- Citrus juice

- Coffee

- Honey

- Maple syrup

- Natural cocoa or chocolate (dark unsweetened varieties from cocoa beans that haven't been 'Dutch-processed' to neutralize their acidity)

- Sour milk (bought from a shop, or made by stirring 1 tsp of vinegar or lemon juice into 1 cup of whole or semi-skimmed milk, and leaving for 15 minutes before using).

- Soured (sour) cream

- Treacle (molasses)

- Vinegar

- Yoghurt

Bicarbonate of soda can also soften dried beans and peas and reduce a food's acidity.

Tips for using bicarbonate of soda

Do

- Store in an airtight container in a cool dry place.

- Sift with other dry ingredients several times before using to ensure thorough mixing.

- Mix ingredients rapidly and cook a mixture without delay to prevent carbon-dioxide bubbles that were released during mixing in the bowl from escaping.

- Use the amount recommended in a recipe. Too little can make a cake rise poorly and the finished product tough and dense. Too much can produce super-size bubbles that make a bread or cake rise too rapidly, which produces a coarse, open-textured loaf or cake and makes fruit and nuts sink. Also, the bursting bubbles make a cake sink in the middle.

- If cooking at high altitude, use less than a recipe suggests, as carbon-dioxide bubbles expand faster when air pressure is relatively low.

- Make chicken skin crispy by rubbing with bicarbonate of soda before cooking.

- If a sauce or casserole tastes too acidic, stir in ½–1 teaspoon of bicarbonate of soda.

- Soak dried beans in water containing bicarbonate of soda. This makes them cook faster, reduces their content of starch and complex carbohydrates, which could ferment in the gut and produce gas, and makes them more digestible. Use 1 teaspoon of bicarbonate of soda for each 200g/7oz/1 cup beans. Soak in a large saucepan of water for 12–24 hours, then rinse and cook.

- Check whether old bicarbonate of soda is usable by mixing ¼ teaspoon with 2 teaspoons of vinegar – it should bubble at once.

Don't

- Add it to green vegetables to retain their colour as they boil, because its alkalinity destroys vitamin C (ascorbic acid).

- Be tempted to use too much, as it could react with fat or oil to form traces of soap, giving the finished product a strange after-taste!

- Substitute it with baking powder, as bicarbonate of soda has four times the raising power.

Baking powder

This contains bicarbonate of soda, two acid-producing compounds, and cornflour (corn starch) – which prolongs its shelf-life by absorbing moisture, thus preventing the premature release of carbon dioxide.

One of the two acid-producing compounds in baking powder is chosen to be fast-acting. This means it produces acid as soon as it combines with water at room temperature in the mixing bowl. Examples include cream of tartar (potassium bitartrate) and calcium acid phosphate (mono-calcium phosphate).

The other acid-producing compound is chosen to be slow-acting. This means it produces acid only when heated in the oven or on the hob. Examples include sodium aluminium sulphate (sodium aluminium sulfate), sodium aluminium phosphate and sodium acid pyrophosphate.

In this way, baking powder produces one batch of bubbles in the mixing bowl and another during cooking. It therefore has a double raising action.

So why don't cooks always use baking powder instead of bicarbonate of soda? First, because many recipes contain an acidic food that will activate sodium bicarbonate. Second, because many recipes don't require a double raising action.

Interestingly, some recipes that call for baking powder still need extra bicarbonate of soda to boost the raising action further, to reduce acidity, to lower the temperature at which sugar caramelizes or to weaken gluten (a cereal-grain-flour protein) to produce a softer cake.

To make baking powder with fast-acting raising ability: put 3 teaspoons of bicarbonate of soda, 4 teaspoons of cream of tartar and 1 teaspoon of cornflour (corn starch) into a jar and shake well.

Tips for using baking powder

- If short of an egg for a cake recipe, add an extra ½ teaspoon of baking powder plus 2 tablespoons of milk.

- Check baking powder is usable by mixing 1 teaspoon with 120ml/4fl oz/½ cup hot water – it should bubble at once. Baking powder has a shelf life of 6–12 months and packs should have a use-by date.

Self-raising flour

Also known as self-rising flour, this is plain (all-purpose) flour combined with baking powder. However, it isn't always a suitable substitute for plain flour plus bicarbonate of soda and an acidic ingredient, such as lemon juice, honey or yoghurt. For example, when making a rich, dense cake, it is better to use plain flour plus baking powder and, perhaps, extra bicarbonate of soda. Some recipes made with self-raising flour also require extra bicarbonate of soda.

To make self-raising flour, for each 450g/1lb/3¾ cups plain flour, add 2 teaspoons of bicarbonate of soda and 4 teaspoons of cream of tartar. Sift three or four times.

Please note:

- Each recipe serves 4.

- 1 tsp (teaspoon) = 5ml; 1 tbsp (tablespoon) = 15ml; 1 cup = 240ml/8fl oz

- All fruit and vegetables are medium-sized unless otherwise stated.

- All eggs are medium (US large) unless otherwise stated.

- If using a fan oven, reduce the temperature recommended in the recipe by 20°C/25°F.

- Please note that salt is included only when needed to cure or soften other ingredients or to enhance their flavour. Anyone who wants to can add salt at the table.

Starters (Appetizers)

Bicarbonate of soda softens dried beans and peas before they are used in such dishes as fried mung beans. In combination with water and an acidic ingredient, it produces bubbles that puff up starchy ingredients such as wheat, polenta (also known as cornmeal or maize meal) or chickpea flour (also known as gram flour, garbanzo flour and besan). This gives us such delights as Hush Puppies (see page 28) and Onion Bhajis (see page 29).

FRIED MUNG BEANS

If you cannot buy split dried mung beans, 'mung dal', to make this snack, use split dried yellow peas instead. Amchoor is ground dried mango.

225g/8oz/1 cup split dried mung beans or yellow peas
1 tsp bicarbonate of soda (baking soda)
olive oil, for frying
1 tbsp lemon juice
½ tsp ground cumin
½ tsp ground ginger
½ tsp ground coriander
½ tsp chilli powder
ground black pepper
½ tsp amchoor (optional)

Put the mung beans into a large bowl of water, add the bicarbonate of soda and soak for 8 hours, topping up with more water if necessary.

Heat plenty of oil in a frying pan (skillet). Fry the beans until whitish and crisp. Remove and drain on kitchen paper. Put them into a bowl and stir in the lemon juice, spices, pepper and ground mango, if using. Serve hot or cold.

HUSH PUPPIES

These savoury Creole corn-batter puffs make a good starter and are great with fish or meat.

oil, for deep-frying
140g/5oz/1 cup polenta
100g/4oz/heaped ¾ cup plain (all-purpose) flour
2 tsp baking powder
1 tsp cayenne pepper
ground black pepper
3 spring onions (scallions), chopped
¼ onion, finely chopped
½ green (bell) pepper, finely chopped
1 egg, beaten
240ml/8fl oz/1 cup milk

Preheat the oil to 190ºC/375ºF. Preheat the oven to 150ºC/300ºF/gas 2.

Put the polenta, flour, baking powder, cayenne pepper and a good grinding of pepper into a large bowl and mix well. Stir in the spring onions, onion and green pepper. Add the beaten egg and half the milk and stir well, then add enough extra milk to form a batter that is stiff but that you can drop from a spoon.

Drop several tablespoons of batter separately into very hot oil and fry for 2–3 minutes or until light golden brown all over, turning them several times as they puff up. Drain on kitchen paper and keep warm in the oven. Cook the remaining batter in batches in the same way.

ONION BHAJIS

Originating in India, these spicy fried balls of onion, spinach and chickpea (gram) flour are popular around the world.

    2 tbsp plain (all-purpose) flour
    1½ tsp bicarbonate of soda
    1 tsp chilli powder (or paprika for milder bhajis)
    ½ tsp ground turmeric
    200g/7oz/scant 2 cups chickpea flour
    50g/2oz/2 cups spinach, chopped
    1 onion, finely chopped
    oil, for deep-frying
    mango chutney or sweet chilli dipping sauce

Sift the plain flour, bicarbonate of soda, chilli and turmeric into a large bowl. Stir in the chickpea flour, spinach and onion. Add enough water to bind the mixture. Leave for 30 minutes.

Heat the oil in a pan until a breadcrumb dropped into it sizzles and browns. Drop in tablespoons of the chickpea mixture and cook, turning occasionally, for 3–4 minutes or until golden-brown.

Remove the bhajis with a slotted spoon and drain on kitchen paper. Serve hot with chutney or sweet chilli dipping sauce.

Vegetables

Bicarbonate of soda helps to soften dried beans and peas before cooking.

MUSHY PEAS

This involves softening dried marrowfat peas overnight in cold water containing a little bicarbonate of soda, then boiling them.

> 2 tsp bicarbonate of soda
> 350g/12oz/heaped 1 cup dried marrowfat peas,
> 30g/1oz/¼ stick butter
> ground black pepper

Soak the peas in a large bowl of water with the bicarbonate of soda for 4–8 hours, or overnight. Drain the peas, rinse under running water, put into a large pan and cover with water. Cover and bring to the boil, then simmer for 1½–2 hours, stirring occasionally.

Drain, then stir in the butter and pepper.

DAL

Also spelt 'daal' and 'dahl', this spicy bean and lentil purée can be scooped up with naan bread (see page 43).

225g/8oz/scant 1 cup dried red kidney beans, soaked overnight in
   water with 1 tsp bicarbonate of soda
175g/6oz/1 cup dried black lentils
3 tbsp oil
2 onions, finely chopped
2 tomatoes, finely chopped
2 garlic cloves, crushed
2.5cm/1in root ginger, grated
1 tsp garam masala
1 tsp chilli powder
1 tsp turmeric
2 tbsp cream
30g/1oz/¼ stick butter
1 large handful coriander (cilantro) leaves, finely chopped

Drain and rinse the kidney beans, then put into a large pan of water, boil for 1¼ hours, then drain. Meanwhile, put the lentils into another pan of water, boil for 30 minutes, then drain.

Heat the oil in a large frying pan (skillet). Add the onions and fry gently until lightly browned. Stir in the tomatoes, garlic and ginger and fry gently for 5 minutes. Stir in the garam masala, chilli powder, turmeric, beans and lentils and fry gently for a further 5 minutes. Stir in the cream, then remove from the heat. Put the butter on top of the dal so it melts, then garnish with coriander.

Main Courses

Batters raised with a leavening agent give us some of our most popular foods. These include waffles, which are a big hit in the US (see page 36), and tempura, which originated in Japan. Bicarbonate of soda is also an important ingredient of falafels, which are particularly popular in North Africa and the Middle East.

FALAFELS

These herb-flavoured delicacies originated in Egypt but are eaten throughout North Africa and in many other countries too. They can also be made from chickpeas.

300g/11oz/2 cups dried broad beans (fava beans)
2 tsp bicarbonate of soda
small handful of dill
small handful of coriander (cilantro) leaves, chopped
small handful of parsley, chopped
½ green (bell) pepper, deseeded and chopped
2 onions, finely chopped
4 garlic cloves, crushed
1 tsp ground cumin
ground black pepper
½ tsp cayenne pepper
1 egg
2 tbsp sesame seeds
oil, for deep-frying
pitta breads and salad, to serve

For the yogurt dip:

400g/14oz/1²/₃ cups natural yogurt

15cm/6in piece of cucumber, chopped

½ onion, chopped

1 garlic clove, crushed

1 tbsp mint leaves, chopped

Soak the beans overnight in a large pan of water containing the bicarbonate of soda. Next morning, put the beans into a large bowl and mash them.

Add the dill, coriander, parsley, green pepper, onions, garlic, cumin, black pepper, cayenne and egg and mix to form a paste. Knead for 2 minutes. Cover with a tea-towel and leave for 30 minutes.

With floured hands, shape a little of the mixture into a ball 4cm/1½in across. Make balls from the remaining mixture. Put the sesame seeds on to a plate and roll each ball in the seeds to coat it.

Heat the oil in a large pan until a cube of bread dropped in sizzles and browns. Deep-fry several balls at a time for 3–4 minutes or until golden brown, turning several times.

Remove the falafels with a slotted spoon and drain on kitchen paper. Repeat with the remaining balls.

Make the yogurt dip by mixing all the ingredients together in a bowl.

Serve the falafels hot or cold with the yoghurt dip, along with pitta breads and salad.

TEMPURA

Tempura batter makes a thin, light and crispy coating for chicken, fish and vegetables. Allow some small lumps of flour to remain, as these give the cooked batter its traditional texture.

75g/3oz/⅔ cup plain (all-purpose) flour, plus extra for dusting

125g/5oz/1 cup cornflour (corn starch)

2 tsp baking powder

ground black pepper

270ml/9fl oz/generous 1 cup ice-cold sparkling water

675g/1lb 8oz chicken breast or fish fillet, cut into 1cm/½in pieces, or 2 aubergines or 4 courgettes (zucchini), cut into 1cm/1½in pieces, or 450g/1lb small mushrooms

oil, for deep-frying

Put the flour, cornflour, baking powder, black pepper and water into a large bowl and mix together lightly.

Heat the olive oil to 190°C/375°F. Dust a few pieces of chicken, fish or vegetable with flour, then lower them into the batter and deep-fry for 2–3 minutes or until light golden brown and crispy. Serve at once.

Desserts and Sweets

Bicarbonate of soda and baking powder come into their own when making sweet treats such as apple fritters, honeycomb and sweet waffles.

APPLE FRITTERS

Pieces of peeled and cored apples coated in a light batter and deep-fried in hot oil make wonderful fritters.

    100g/4oz/heaped ¾ cup plain (all-purpose) flour
    1 tsp ground cinnamon
    1 tbsp olive oil
    1 egg, separated
    about 70ml/2½ fl oz/⅓ cup milk
    1 tsp baking powder
    4 large eating apples (sweet dessert apples), peeled, cored and
        cut into 6mm/¼in rings or slices
    oil, for deep-frying
    caster (superfine) sugar, to sprinkle
    vanilla ice cream, to serve

Sift the flour and cinnamon into a bowl. Stir in the olive oil, egg yolk and enough milk to make a batter that just coats the back of a wooden spoon. Leave for half an hour. Immediately before using it, whisk the egg white. Then stir the baking powder into the batter and fold in the whisked egg white.

Heat the oil to 190°C/375°F. Dip a few apple rings or slices into the batter then drop them into the hot oil. Turn them several times, and when golden-brown remove with a slotted spoon and drain on kitchen paper. Repeat with the remaining pieces of apple.

Sprinkle with sugar and serve warm with vanilla ice cream.

Tips:

- For a spicy batter, add 1 teaspoon of ground cinnamon to the flour.

- Ring the changes with slices of fresh or tinned pineapple, or bananas cut into 5cm/2in chunks instead of apple.

WAFFLES

To make these vanilla-flavoured waffles, you will need to use a waffle iron that you heat on the hob, or an electric waffle iron.

If you would prefer unsweetened waffles to eat with bacon and scrambled egg or grated cheese, omit the sugar and vanilla.

100g/4oz/heaped ¾ cup plain (all-purpose) flour

2 tsp baking powder

2 tbsp caster (superfine) sugar

1 egg, separated

30g/1oz/¼ stick unsalted butter, melted, plus extra for greasing

½ tsp vanilla extract

about 240ml/8fl oz/1 cup milk

maple syrup, golden syrup, jam, butter or ice cream, to serve

Sift the flour and baking powder into a large bowl and stir in the sugar. Make a well in the centre and drop in the egg yolk, melted butter and vanilla essence. Gradually beat in enough of the milk to make a smooth batter with the consistency of thin cream. Whisk the egg white until stiff, then fold it into the batter. Pour the batter into a measuring jug.

Heat the waffle iron, brush it with melted butter, heat it again, then fill one side with enough waffle batter to reach the top without overflowing. Cook the waffles for around half a minute or until golden-brown on both sides. Remove the waffles and serve warm with maple syrup, golden syrup, jam, butter or ice cream.

Use the remaining batter to make more waffles, each time brushing any debris from the waffle iron and re-greasing it.

Cakes and Biscuits

Almost every cake recipe contains bicarbonate of soda either as the sole raising agent or in baking powder.

SEMOLINA CAKES

These cakes, made with semolina and soaked in syrup or honey, have a very long history in India, Pakistan, Bangladesh, Afghanistan, Iran and Greece, Turkey and other Mediterranean countries. They are also known as 'semolina halva', and their distinctive and delightful texture is less dense than that of halva made with tahini (sesame-paste).

115g/4oz/1 stick butter

50g/2oz/¼ cup caster (superfine) sugar

1 tsp vanilla extract

2 eggs, beaten

175g/6oz/¾ cup plain yoghurt

400g/14oz/3⅓ cups semolina

1 tsp baking powder

½ tsp bicarbonate of soda

12 blanched split almonds

For the syrup:

400g/14oz/scant 2 cups granulated sugar

1 tbsp lemon juice

Preheat the oven to 180ºC/350ºF/gas 4. Grease a 20 x 30cm/8 x 12in shallow baking tin (pan).

Put the butter, sugar and vanilla essence into a large bowl and beat well until light and creamy in colour. Beat in the eggs one at a time, then add a little of the yoghurt.

Sift the semolina, baking powder and bicarbonate of soda twice into another large bowl. Fold this into the egg mixture a little at a time, alternating with the remaining yoghurt. Pour the mixture into the baking tin and decorate with rows of almonds on top. Bake for 30–35 minutes or until a skewer inserted into the cake comes out clean.

To make the syrup, put the sugar, lemon juice and 350ml/12fl oz/ scant 1½ cups water into a small saucepan. Bring to the boil, stirring constantly, and boil rapidly for 10 minutes. Remove from the heat and cool the pan by standing it in cold water.

Once the cake is cooked, spoon the cooled syrup over it. Once cold, cut it into diamonds or squares.

CIDER CAKE

The cider in this recipe is just acidic enough to activate the bicarbonate of soda. This produces bubbles of carbon dioxide, which make the cake rise.

225g/8oz/scant 2 cups plain (all-purpose) flour
1 tsp bicarbonate of soda
1 tsp ground nutmeg
100g/4oz/1 stick butter, softened, plus extra for greasing
100g/4oz/scant ½ cup caster (superfine) sugar
2 eggs, beaten
150ml/5fl oz/generous ½ cup sweet cider (sweet apple cider)

Preheat the oven to 180°C/350°F/gas 4. Grease an 18cm/7in square baking tin (pan).

Sift the flour, bicarbonate of soda and nutmeg into a bowl.

Put the butter and sugar into a large bowl and beat with a wooden spoon until smooth and pale. Add 1 tablespoon of the beaten eggs and 1 tablespoon of the flour mixture and beat well. Repeat, then beat in the remaining beaten egg.

Add the remaining flour mixture and stir well. Then add the cider and beat the mixture until it begins to froth.

Pour into the tin and bake for 40 minutes or until the cake shrinks from the sides of the tin. Turn out on to a wire rack to cool.

DEVIL'S FOOD CAKE

Bicarbonate of soda reddens natural cocoa (which is slightly acidic) during baking, hence the name 'devil's food cake'. Natural cocoa powder is neither Dutch-processed (treated with an alkali to neutralize the acids) nor sweetened. You can also produce a fine cake with Dutched cocoa powder as long as the recipe contains an acidic ingredient such as coffee (as below). Note that it doesn't matter what type of milk you use.

100g/4oz/1 stick unsalted butter, at room temperature, plus extra
    for greasing
150g/5oz/1¼ cups plain (all-purpose) flour
75g/2½oz/scant ⅔ cup cocoa powder, preferably natural
1 tsp bicarbonate of soda
¼ tsp baking powder
120ml/4fl oz/½ cup strong coffee
120ml/4fl oz/½ cup milk
340g/12oz/1½ cups granulated sugar
2 large (extra large) eggs, at room temperature

For the frosting:
275g/10oz/10 squares dark (semisweet) chocolate, coarsely
    chopped
150g/5oz/1½ sticks unsalted butter, finely chopped

Preheat the oven to 180°C/350°F/gas 4. Grease and line two 23cm/9in round cake tins (pans).

Sift the flour, cocoa powder, bicarbonate of soda and baking powder into a large bowl. Put the coffee and milk into a small bowl and stir well.

Put the butter and sugar into another large bowl and beat with a wooden spoon for at least 5 minutes, until light and creamy. Alternatively, do this with a standing electric mixer. Add one of the eggs and a tablespoon of the flour mixture and beat well. Repeat with the other egg.

Stir in half the flour mixture, then the coffee and milk mixture, then the remaining flour mixture. Pour the batter into the tins and bake for 25 minutes or until a skewer inserted into the middle comes out clean. Leave to cool for a few minutes, then turn out on to a wire rack and leave to cool completely.

To make the frosting, melt the chocolate and 120ml/4fl oz/½ cup water in a bowl over a pan of simmering water, stirring occasionally. Remove from the heat, add the butter and stir until melted. Leave to cool for 1 hour or until the frosting is thick enough to be spread.

Place one cake on a plate and spread a third of the frosting on top. Place the other cake on top and spread the top and sides of the whole cake with the remaining frosting.

GINGERBREAD MEN

In Scandinavian countries it is traditional to make these biscuits in the run-up to Christmas.

225g/8oz/²/₃ cup golden syrup
150g/5oz/scant ¾ cup granulated sugar
1 tsp ground ginger
1 tsp ground cinnamon
1 tsp ground cloves
150g/5oz/1¼ sticks butter
1½ tsp bicarbonate of soda
1 egg, beaten
550g/1lb 4oz/4¼ cups plain (all-purpose) flour, plus extra for
    dusting
glacé icing to decorate (optional)

Put the syrup, sugar, spices and butter into a large saucepan and heat gently, stirring, until the sugar and butter have melted. Leave to cool for 15 minutes. Dissolve the bicarbonate of soda in 2 teaspoons water and add to the pan. Add the egg, sift in the flour and mix together.

Transfer the resulting dough to a bowl and leave in a cool place for 1 hour to make it easier to roll out.

Preheat the oven to 220ºC/425ºF/gas 7. Grease 4 baking (cookie) sheets.

Put the dough on a floured board and roll to about 3mm/⅛in thick. Cut out about 20 shapes, depending on size, with gingerbread-man or other cookie cutters and put them on the baking sheets.

Bake for 10–15 minutes until golden brown. Loosen with a palette knife, then transfer to wire racks to cool. Decorate with glacé icing, if wanted.

Breads, Oatcakes and Scones

Bicarbonate of soda makes a rapid-acting alternative to yeast as a raising agent for breads and scones and also avoids ending up with a yeasty flavour.

NAAN BREAD

This flat bread is a staple in South and Central Asia and is wonderful for mopping up sauces.

    250g/9oz/heaped 2 cups plain or wholemeal (wholegrain) flour,
        plus extra for dusting
    2 tsp caster (superfine) sugar
    ½ tsp baking powder
    ½ tsp bicarbonate of soda
    120ml/4fl oz/½ cup milk
    2 tbsp olive oil, plus extra for greasing
    3 tbsp yoghurt
    2 garlic cloves, chopped and lightly fried in a little oil or butter
        (optional)
    1 tbsp coriander (cilantro) leaves, chopped (optional)
    2oz/50g/⅓ cup poppy or sesame seeds (optional)
    15g/½oz/1 tbsp butter, melted

Sift the flour, sugar, baking powder and bicarbonate of soda into a large bowl and make a well in the centre. Pour the milk, oil and yoghurt into another bowl and stir well, then pour this mixture into the well. Add the garlic or coriander, if using.

Turn the mixture out onto a floured surface and knead for 10 minutes, adding a little more flour if the dough is too sticky.

Put the dough into a greased bowl, cover with a damp tea towel and leave in a warm place for 2–3 hours. Shape into five balls.

Preheat the oven to 220°C/425°F/gas 7. Put two baking (cookie) sheets into the oven to heat up.

Roll out the dough balls thinly into teardrop shapes. Sprinkle poppy or sesame seeds on to the flattened dough shapes, if using, and press into their surface.

Put the breads on the hot baking sheets and bake for about 10 minutes or until slightly puffed up and light golden brown.

Pour the melted butter over the naan breads and serve hot.

Variation: **Peshwari naans**

> 4 tsp caster (superfine) sugar
>
> 2 tbsp ground almonds (optional)
>
> 1 tbsp desiccated coconut, soaked in water then squeezed out (optional)
>
> 2 tbsp sultanas (golden raisins)

For sweet Peshwari naans, make the naan dough as above, then mix the sugar, ground almonds (if using), coconut (if using) and sultanas together. Slightly flatten each dough ball, put some filling into the centre, then bring the sides over the mixture to stick together in the middle. Roll into shapes gently so that the filling does not spill out. Cook as above.

CORN BREAD

Traditional in the southern states of the US, this bread, with its light and gritty texture from the polenta (also known as cornmeal and maize meal), looks like a tray-bake. When combined with onions and sage gently fried in butter, it also makes an excellent stuffing (dressing) for a turkey.

100g/4oz/1 stick butter, melted, plus extra for greasing
175g/6oz/1½ cups plain (all-purpose) flour
1 tbsp baking powder
275g/10oz/scant 2 cups polenta
2 tbsp caster (superfine) sugar
4 eggs, beaten
240ml/8fl oz/1 cup milk
50ml/2fl oz/scant ¼ cup single ('half and half') cream

Preheat the oven to 200°C/400°F/gas 6. Grease a 20cm/8in square heavy baking dish and put it in the oven.

Sift the flour and baking powder into a large bowl. Stir in the polenta and sugar. Pour in the butter and stir until the mixture resembles breadcrumbs.

Put the eggs and milk into another bowl and whisk. Stir into the flour and butter mixture. Then stir in the cream to make a paste-like mixture.

Take the warmed baking dish from the oven and spoon in the mixture. Bake for 25–30 minutes or until a skewer inserted into the centre comes out clean. Leave to cool for 5 minutes. Serve hot or cold in large squares or slices.

IRISH SODA BREAD

This was the first recipe I learnt at school from our cookery teacher –
a red-haired woman called Mrs Stallebrass. She said it was quicker to
cook than yeast-raised bread, so if we could make it we'd never be short
of bread for unexpected guests. Soda bread originated in Ireland, and
in south-west Ireland it is often called 'cake'. Eat the bread with butter
and jam, or soup, or use it to mop up gravy or another sauce.

> 400g/14oz/2¾ cups wholemeal (wholegrain) flour
> 100g/4oz/heaped ¾ cup plain (all-purpose) flour
> 60g/2½oz/scant ½ cup polenta (cornmeal)
> 1 tsp bicarbonate of soda
> 480–720ml/16–24fl oz/2–3 cups buttermilk (or milk plus an
>   extra ½ tsp baking powder)

Preheat the oven to 230ºC/450ºF/gas 8. Dust a baking (cookie) sheet
with flour. Sift the flours, polenta and bicarbonate of soda into a large
bowl. Make a well in the centre and quickly stir in three-quarters of
the buttermilk, adding more if necessary to make a very soft, even
slightly sticky dough. Put this on to a floured surface and knead quickly
(any longer would allow carbon-dioxide bubbles to escape and thereby
toughen the bread).

Put the dough on to the baking sheet and shape into a mound
15–20cm/6–8in in diameter. With a knife mark a cross across the top;
the cuts should go halfway down the sides so the loaf will 'flower' as
the dough expands in the oven.

Bake for 10 minutes, then reduce the heat to 200ºC/400ºF/gas 6
and bake for another 35 minutes. For a crunchy crust, cool on a rack
uncovered; for a softer crust, wrap the loaf in a damp tea towel.

OATCAKES

These biscuits (crackers) are delicious with cheese or jam. Note that oatmeal is made by grinding whole dehusked oats to a fine, medium or coarse grade of meal. Steelcut oats are made by cutting rolled oats, and rolled oats are made by rolling whole oats, but neither type has a suitable texture for this recipe. In the US a coarse 'Scottish' oatmeal, available online from www.bobsredmill.com, will produce a coarse-textured oatcake. However, you can whizz it in a food processor for a short time to make its texture approximate that of medium oatmeal.

75g/3oz/scant ⅔ cup self-raising (self-rising) flour
100g/4oz/heaped ¾ cup medium oatmeal
½ tsp baking powder
50g/2oz/4 tbsp white vegetable shortening
flour, for dusting

Preheat the oven to 200ºC/400ºF/gas 6. Grease a baking (cookie) sheet.

Put the flour, oatmeal and baking powder into a large bowl and mix well. Lightly rub in (cut in) the vegetable shortening until the mixture is crumbly. Gradually add enough cold water to form a stiff dough.

Put the dough on to a lightly floured surface and roll it out to 5mm/¼in thick. Use a large round plain cutter (or a teacup) to form 8–10 circles. Put these on to the baking sheet and bake for about 20 minutes, taking care that the oatcakes do not brown. Transfer to a wire rack to cool.

SCONES

Warm scones with butter and jam are a treat fit for the gods. Some people also enjoy them with cheese and chutney. If you want to make buttermilk scones, omit the cream of tartar.

30g/1oz/¼ stick chilled butter, diced, plus extra for greasing
225g/8oz/scant 2 cups plain (all-purpose) flour, plus extra for
  dusting
1 tsp bicarbonate of soda
2 tsp cream of tartar (optional)
50g/2oz/scant ½ cup sultanas (golden raisins) (optional)
about 150ml/5fl oz/generous ½ cup milk or buttermilk

Preheat the oven to 230°C/450°F/gas 8. Lightly grease a baking sheet.

Sift the flour, bicarbonate of soda and cream of tartar (if using) into a large bowl and lightly rub in (cut in) the butter. Stir in the sultanas (if using). Immediately mix in enough of the milk or buttermilk to make a soft dough, using a round-bladed knife.

Turn the dough out on to a lightly floured surface and knead the dough quickly until smooth. Roll it out to 2cm/¾in thick and cut out 8–10 rounds with a 5cm/2in cutter. Place on a baking (cookie) sheet and brush the tops with milk.

Bake the scones for about 10 minutes, until well risen and golden brown. Transfer to a wire rack to cool.

SINGING HINNIES

These fried scones are teatime treats that originated in the north of England. Affectionately known as 'hinnies' ('hinny' is Geordie for 'honey'), they delight the ear by whistling or 'singing' as they cook.

225g/8oz/scant 2 cups plain (all-purpose) flour
50g/2oz/½ stick butter, plus extra for frying
50g/2oz/4 tbsp white vegetable shortening
30g/1oz/¼ cup currants
1 tsp baking powder
about 2 tbsp milk

Put the flour, butter and shortening into a large bowl and rub in (cut in) the fats until the mixture resembles fine breadcrumbs. Add the currants, baking powder and milk and stir to form a soft dough.

Roll the dough out on a floured surface to form a circle about 2cm/¾in thick. Cut into 6–8 wedges.

Melt some butter in a large frying pan (skillet), reduce the heat and cook the circle of wedges on both sides until lightly browned.

Split and serve with butter and jam or golden syrup.

SCOTCH PANCAKES

These small thick pancakes are made from a thick pancake batter puffed up a little with bicarbonate of soda. Their other name is 'drop scones'. Buttermilk is a good alternative to the milk, but if using this you should halve the amount of cream of tartar.

225g/8oz/scant 2 cups plain (all-purpose) flour
1 tsp bicarbonate of soda
1 tsp cream of tartar
75g/3oz/⅓ cup caster (superfine) sugar
2 eggs
300ml/10½fl oz/1¼ cups milk
butter, for frying

Sift the flour, bicarbonate of soda and cream of tartar into a large bowl. Stir in the sugar. Make a well in the centre and whisk in the eggs and enough milk to make a smooth batter.

Melt a knob of butter in a frying pan (skillet) or on a griddle. Spoon tablespoonfuls of batter into the pan, leaving enough room for them to spread. When the pancakes puff up and bubbles start bursting on their surface, turn them over with a palette knife. Cook until golden-brown underneath.

Remove the pancakes from the heat, place them on a tea towel and cover with another tea towel to keep them warm and prevent them drying out while you cook the next batch.

CHAPTER 3

Beauty and personal care

Bicarbonate of soda (baking soda) is a great beauty aid and is also useful for other personal care.

For one thing, it softens water, so you need less soap to wash your face and body and less shampoo to wash your hair. This is good because the more soap or shampoo you use, the more you strip valuable natural oils and acidity from your skin and scalp.

For another, its very mildly abrasive nature means that it helps to clean the skin. Its tiny rounded particles also have gentle exfoliating properties, helping to dislodge dead cells. This smoothes and brightens skin, making it look younger and healthier. What's more, it stimulates the skin's tiny blood vessels (capillaries), giving the skin a soft attractive glow. It can also help to clear blackheads.

When present in toothpaste, bicarbonate of soda can help to remove dental plaque (the sticky film of food residues and bacteria that accumulates on teeth) and tartar (hard, calcium-impregnated plaque that encourages gum disease). Its alkalinity is helpful for teeth, too. For example, it can neutralize the acidity released during the breakdown of sugars and other refined carbohydrates by mouth bacteria. This is important, because acidity encourages teeth to decay.

Bicarbonate of soda's alkalinity has antiseptic and antifungal actions that can help to prevent or treat minor skin and scalp infections. It also has a deodorant action that is thought to result from neutralization of odoriferous short-chain fatty acids in the sweat produced in the armpits, for example.

Finally, bicarbonate of soda is a common ingredient in the effervescent balls of bath salts known as 'bath bombs'.

Here you'll find tips for using bicarbonate for personal care, as well as bicarbonate-containing recipes for toiletries such as toothpaste, deodorant and 'bath bombs'.

Bathing

To soften bathwater add 100g/3½oz/½ cup bicarbonate of soda to your bath. A few drops of fragrant oil will make your bath-time particularly sybaritic. Cedarwood, frankincense and lavender essential oils are said to be relaxing, while geranium, jasmine, neroli and ylang ylang are considered uplifting, and cardamom stimulating and refreshing.

For extra cleaning power, so you don't need to use soap, add several squeezes of shampoo.

For a seaside-spa-style bath, add 300g/3½oz/½ cup bicarbonate of soda plus 100g/4oz/½ cup sea salt to the water.

To make 'bath bombs' (colourful fragrant lumps of bath salts that fizz when added to bath water), mix 200g/14oz/2 cups bicarbonate of soda and 200g/7oz/1 cup citric acid (from a pharmacy or the internet) together in a bowl. Add 10 drops of fragrant essential oil plus a few drops of food colouring. Now add about 1 teaspoon of almond oil or baby oil, a few drops at a time, until the mixture is crumbly but just clumps together when firmly squeezed. Firmly press it into moulds such as plastic egg boxes, silicone or other non-stick fairy-cake moulds, little yoghurt pots, or special moulds from craft stores. Leave to dry for a week. Then, when you have a bath, put a 'bath bomb' in the water and watch it fizz as its citric acid and bicarbonate of soda react with the water to release bubbles of carbon dioxide.

Washing-up

If you dislike wearing rubber gloves, help to keep your hands soft by adding 1 tablespoon of bicarbonate of soda to the washing-up water.

Deodorizing

- Adding bicarbonate of soda to your bath water (see 'Bathing', opposite) will help to keep you odour-free.

- In a small bowl, mix ½ teaspoon of bicarbonate of soda, 1 or 2 drops of water and, if required, 1 drop of fragrant essential oil. Smooth a little of this deodorant paste under your arms.

- Alternatively, pat on bicarbonate of soda as a dry deodorant.

- Sprinkle bicarbonate of soda between toes, or into tights (pantyhose) or socks, as an alternative to talcum powder to help keep feet fresh and dry.

- Shake a little bicarbonate of soda on a new sanitary pad before use.

Exfoliating

- After cleansing your skin, make an exfoliant paste by mixing about 3 parts of bicarbonate of soda to 1 part of water. Gently rub this into your skin, then rinse off.

- To smooth roughened lips, rub them with a paste made by mixing bicarbonate of soda with lemon juice. Rinse and then apply some lip balm.

- Smooth cuticles by wetting them, rubbing in a little bicarbonate of soda, then rinsing, drying and applying moisturizer.

Softening dry, rough or hard skin

Make a skin-softening paste by combining bicarbonate of soda and extra-virgin olive oil. Add fragrance, if you like, by adding a few drops of lavender, rose or neroli essential oil. Smooth the paste over your hands, elbows, the bottoms of your feet or other areas of dry, rough or hard skin. Wait for 30 minutes then rinse off the paste with warm water and immediately smooth in some moisturizing cream.

Shaving

- Mix bicarbonate of soda with water to form a loose paste and apply this to your skin before shaving as an alternative to soap lather or shaving cream or gel. This is less 'drying' to the skin than most soaps because it doesn't reduce the skin's natural oils and acidity.

- Quickly soothe a shaving rash by smoothing on a paste made from bicarbonate of soda and water, as above. You can wash the paste off visible areas such as your face or legs before you see other people.

- Help to prevent a shaving rash by smoothing on a paste made from bicarbonate of soda and water, as above.

Clearing blackheads

Twice a day, clean and dry your face. In a small bowl, mix 1 tablespoon of bicarbonate of soda with about 1 teaspoon of water to make a paste. Rub this over your skin to help loosen and remove blackheads, leave for 10–20 minutes, then rinse. Now help to restore your skin's natural acidity by patting on a little cider vinegar (apple cider vinegar).

Hair-care

Remove a build-up of products, such as hairsprays and hair gels, by squeezing your usual amount of shampoo into the palm of your hand and mixing in 1–2 teaspoons of bicarbonate of soda. Use this to wash your hair, then rinse well. Repeat, then condition your hair.

Dry-clean greasy hair when short of time by sprinkling it with bicarbonate of soda, rubbing this through with your hands, then brushing thoroughly.

Dental care

Coat your toothbrush bristles with bicarbonate of soda before brushing your teeth. This 'dry-brushing' with bicarbonate removes plaque better than 'wet-brushing'. Bicarbonate of soda cleans and brightens teeth. It also counteracts the acidity that is produced by mouth bacteria from traces of sugars and other refined carbohydrates, and which encourages tooth decay.

Some people advocate making a fresher-tasting paste by mixing equal amounts of bicarbonate of soda and fine sea salt. Salt boosts the flow of saliva (which has anti-bacterial properties, so helping prevent tooth decay) and contains the alkaline mineral sodium, which helps to counteract acidity.

Make a whitening toothpaste by mixing bicarbonate of soda with 3 per cent hydrogen peroxide solution. Use it once a week and rinse your mouth thoroughly with water afterwards. Hydrogen peroxide is available from certain pharmacies (drugstores).

Make a cleansing, refreshing mouthwash by mixing ½ teaspoon bicarbonate of soda in ¼ glass of warm water. Take a mouthful and swish it around your mouth.

Foot-care

Soothe aching feet by adding 4 tablespoons of bicarbonate of soda to a washing-up bowl of warm water. Put this on the floor, sit on a chair and soak your feet for 10–15 minutes. Add several drops of essential oil for fragrance (for suggested choices, see the first tip in 'Bathing', page 52).

CHAPTER 4

Your body's bicarbonate

Good health (and, indeed, life itself) relies on our blood and other body fluids having the right acid–alkali balance. The bicarbonate that is naturally present in our body helps this to happen.

There is a lot of scientific information in this chapter, but, as the poet TS Eliot said, 'Wisdom may be lost in information', so if you prefer to skip the science, you'll find practical ways of correcting an acid–alkali imbalance in the next two chapters. Note that if do you decide to read this chapter, there is a glossary explaining many of the technical terms at the end (see page 76).

Where does the bicarbonate in our body come from?

The building blocks of our body's bicarbonate originate from food and drink:

- As our cells produce energy from sugar (which is mainly derived from dietary carbohydrate), they release carbon dioxide. This can react reversibly with water to form carbonic acid – a weak acid that breaks down reversibly into bicarbonate and hydrogen.

- Many foods contain carbonates or other organic substances that the body can convert into bicarbonate. ('Organic' is used here in its chemical sense, meaning these substances contain only carbon, oxygen and, perhaps, hydrogen.)

- Any bicarbonate consumed in food or drink neutralizes a certain amount of stomach acid; any excess is absorbed from the intestine into the blood.

Some people also get bicarbonate from antacids or other medications.

Body fluids

Fluid accounts for nearly 60 per cent of the weight of a man's body and 55 per cent of a woman's. The average man's body, weighing 70kg/154lb, contains 42 litres/74 pints/89 US pints, comprising:

- 25 litres/44 pints/53 US pints of intracellular fluid (fluid in cells).

- 17 litres/30 pints/36 US pints of extracellular fluid (fluid outside cells), including:

  - 11.5 litres/20 pints/24 US pints of tissue fluid (fluid that bathes cells)

  - 5 litres/9 pints/10.5 US pints of blood (circulating in blood vessels)

  - 500ml/17fl oz/2 cups of other extracellular fluids (including

lymph, bile, saliva, pancreatic juice, spinal fluid, joint fluid
and eye fluid).

Acid–alkali balance

Each body fluid is a watery solution containing electrolytes (substances
that can break down into electrically charged particles called ions). A
fluid is said to be *acidic* if its concentration of hydrogen ions is greater
than that of its hydroxyl ions, and *alkaline* if the other way around.

One hydrogen ion and one hydroxide ion can combine to form a
molecule of water. A solution is *neutral* (neither acidic nor alkaline) if
its hydrogen and hydroxide-ion concentrations are equal.

Our body's acids include:

- Carbonic acid. This is called a 'volatile' acid because it can break
  down into carbon dioxide and water, which can be breathed out
  by the lungs.

- Strong inorganic acidic anions, including chloride (from the
  breakdown of dietary proteins) and sulphate (sulfate) (made
  from dietary proteins by the breakdown of the sulphur (sulfur)-
  containing amino acids methionine and cysteine).

- Weak inorganic acidic anions, mainly phosphate (from the
  breakdown of dietary proteins) and albumin (a blood protein
  made by the liver) but also nitrate and the amino acid glutamine
  (from dietary proteins), and other blood proteins.

- Organic acidic anions, including lactate, pyruvate, malate,
  formate and ketones, made by our cells.

What is pH and why is it important?

A body fluid's pH ('potential of Hydrogen') represents its hydrogen-ion concentration, which in turn indicates its acid–alkali balance. Each number on the pH scale represents a ten-fold decrease in hydrogen-ion concentration from the one below and a ten-fold increase from the one above.

- A fluid becomes more acidic as its hydrogen-ion concentration rises and its pH falls, and becomes more alkaline as its hydrogen-ion concentration falls and its pH rises.

- The pH scale goes from 0 to 14, with 7 neutral for water. Because pH is temperature-dependent, a neutral pH for blood at body temperature would be 6.7. But we would die if it were neutral! It must always be alkaline. And it must stay within a very small range of pH.

The pH of body fluids

Most body fluids are alkaline. Their pHs are regulated by our lungs, kidneys and buffers (see page 64). And they affect each other in various important ways.

- Normal arterial blood and tissue fluid have an average alkaline pH of 7.4 (range 7.35–7.45). Venous blood is slightly less alkaline at 7.36 (since cells produce acids, releasing hydrogen ions that can enter veins).

- Intracellular fluid has a pH of about 7.

- Pancreatic juice is particularly alkaline at pH 7.5–8.8. Urine can be acidic or alkaline (pH 4.5–7.5). Stomach juice is very acidic (pH 1–2). As stomach contents enter the duodenum (the first part of the small intestine), they are alkalinized by bile and pancreatic juice. The skin's surface moisture, from skin oil and sweat, mostly has a pH of 4.5–5.75, but is slightly less acidic in the armpits and around the genitals.

Does a change in pH matter?

A change in the pHs of blood, tissue fluid or intracellular fluid can have vitally important consequences to our health, wellbeing and even life itself, by affecting:

- Energy production (measurable as a person's 'basal metabolic rate')

- Molecular reactivity

- Bonding of oxygen and carbon dioxide to haemoglobin (the pigment in red blood cells) and therefore the transport of oxygen to cells and carbon dioxide from cells

- Oxidation (a low pH encourages the production of 'free radicals' – also known as reactive oxygen-containing ions)

- Muscle-cell contraction

- Enzyme activity

- 'Folding', and therefore function, of proteins (including structural ones)

- Exchange of potassium and sodium across cell membranes

- Bio-electric signalling in and between cells

- Calcium balance

- Fatty acid and cholesterol metabolism

- Levels and activity of, and sensitivity to, certain hormones (for example, adrenaline, thyroxine and growth hormone)

- Cell growth, differentiation, multiplication and apoptosis ('cell suicide')

- Cell mobility

- Behaviour of red blood cells (a low pH makes them stack up so that they cannot properly transport oxygen, carbon dioxide, nutrients and waste products)

- Size and behaviour of white cells (a low pH makes them smaller and less active)

The degree of pH change required to affect cells isn't always clear. However, a very abnormal pH (below 6.8 or above 7.8) makes the normal folded shape of each protein molecule begin to 'unravel'. If this continues, life continues for only a few hours.

How the body responds to changes in pH

When the body-fluids' normal pHs are threatened or actually changed by diet, lifestyle, disease or medication, the following things happen:

- Lungs exhale more carbon dioxide to reduce acidity, or less to increase acidity.

- Kidneys excrete more strong inorganic acidic anions (mainly chloride) to reduce acidity, or fewer to increase acidity. This pH-regulation is slower than that of the lungs.

- Body fluids buffer (minimize) pH changes by changing the levels of bicarbonate, non-volatile weak inorganic acidic ions or acids.

- Liver can metabolize organic acidic anions (for example, it converts lactate into glycogen).

- Cell membranes allow a greater or smaller passage of various ions between cells, tissue fluid and blood.

- Sympathetic nervous system produces more or less adrenaline to stimulate the heart, lungs and kidneys.

- Sweat contains more or fewer acidic anions (such as phosphates, sulphates, chlorides and lactates).

- The above responses affect the following independent pH-regulating factors in body fluids:

    1. Strong-ion difference. Most body fluids are alkaline because their concentration of strong alkaline cations (sodium, potassium and, to a lesser extent, calcium and magnesium) is greater than that of strong acidic anions (chloride, sulphate, phosphate, lactate). The strong-ion difference and, therefore, the pH, fall with a decrease in strong cations or an increase in strong anions, and vice versa. The strong-ion difference is affected by our diet and the activity of our digestive tract, kidneys and cells.

    2. Carbon dioxide. This flows from cells to tissue fluid to blood. It can also flow the other way. The amount in our body fluids varies with changes in metabolism, circulation and breathing rate.

    3. Non-volatile weak inorganic acids.

Changes in the above factors in turn change our bicarbonate and hydrogen-ion levels.

Bicarbonate and the lungs

Carbon dioxide produced by cell metabolism is carried in the blood to the lungs, where any excess is breathed out to prevent it reducing our blood pH (and so making it less alkaline).

If something threatens to lower our blood pH, we automatically breathe more rapidly and exhale more carbon dioxide, and vice versa.

Bicarbonate and the kidneys

Our kidneys filter bicarbonate from the blood and excrete about 20 per cent of it. If something threatens to lower our blood pH, the kidneys excrete less bicarbonate, and vice versa.

Bicarbonate buffer

Buffers change their concentration to help maintain the body's acid–alkali balance. Bicarbonate is our most important buffer. Bicarbonate ions can raise pH (thereby increasing alkalinity) by joining with hydrogen ions to form carbonic acid.

Carbonic acid can lower pH (thereby reducing alkalinity) by breaking down into hydrogen and bicarbonate ions. Carbonic acid is such a weak acid that in itself it has negligible acidity.

Acidosis and alkalosis

Acidosis is a 'push' towards acidity, or, more accurately (because blood, tissue fluid and intracellular fluid are never actually acidic), a push towards lowered alkalinity. This is associated with the accumulation of acid and hydrogen ions, or loss of bicarbonate.

The lungs, kidneys and buffers try to compensate so as to maintain or restore a normal blood pH. While this is perfectly normal, if prolonged or extreme it can 'strain' the body and cause symptoms. Depending on the success of compensation, the blood pH either remains within its normal range or falls below 7.35 (which causes symptoms – see below).

Alkalosis is a 'push' towards over-alkalinity. The lungs, kidneys and buffers try to compensate for this. Depending on their success, the blood pH may remain within its normal range or rise above 7.45. Alkalosis is much less common than acidosis.

Lactic acidosis

However, acidosis isn't all bad. For example, lactic acidosis associated with lactate production in muscle cells during strenuous exercise increases the oxygen available to them.

Certain people's cells oxidize sugar (to produce energy) particularly rapidly. This encourages lactic acidosis. Such people are known as 'fast oxidizers' and tend to feel hungry after a meal sooner than do others.

Note that:

- Symptoms from acidosis or alkalosis result from changes in blood, tissue fluid and intracellular fluid of the levels of strong ions (such as sodium, potassium, chloride and sulphate); the amount of carbon dioxide; and the concentration of non-volatile weak inorganic acids. Changes in these independent pH-regulating factors are accompanied by changes in levels of hydrogen and bicarbonate ions.

- It is vital to try to identify and treat the underlying cause.
- The causes of acidosis and alkalosis are metabolic, respiratory or mixed.

The following lists are based on acidosis below pH 7.35 ('acidemia') and alkalosis above pH 7.45 ('alkalemia'). But certain causes, symptoms and treatments also pertain to less severe acidosis or alkalosis.

Metabolic acidosis

This results from a build-up of acids from an acid-forming diet, increased acid production, reduced acid excretion or loss of alkali. There may also be too much chloride. The causes include:

1. Lactic acidosis from increased or impaired energy production in cells, resulting from:

    - strenuous exercise

    - severe infection

    - prolonged or widespread inflammation

    - prolonged lack of oxygen, for example, from a seizure, severe anaemia, shock, lung disease, heart failure

    - too much alcohol, especially if a person lacks vitamin B1

- low blood sugar, which increases adrenaline (so as to increase blood sugar) and thereby speeds muscle-cell metabolism

- prolonged stress, anxiety or anger, as this increases adrenaline

- smoking

- certain drugs including metformin (for diabetes)

- liver failure

- certain cancers (such as lymphoma and leukaemia).

2. Uncontrolled diabetes, a low-carbohydrate diet or starvation, which means that fats are used instead of sugar for energy, producing acidic substances called ketones.

3. Aspirin and certain other medications.

4. Severe diarrhoea originating in the small intestine and causing a loss of bicarbonate, or the genetic kidney disease proximal renal tubular acidosis, which causes a loss of bicarbonate in urine or the retention of hydrogen ions, or both.

5. Kidney failure or distal renal tubular acidosis, which reduce urinary excretion of acidic sulphates, phosphates and urates.

6. An acid-forming diet and an age-related decline in kidney function, though these cannot in themselves reduce the pH below 7.3.

What happens? The lungs try to compensate with deep rapid breathing that reduces the blood's level of carbon dioxide. The kidneys try to compensate by excreting more hydrogen and less bicarbonate.

Symptoms: headache, anxiety, drowsiness, fatigue, poor vision, nausea, vomiting, abdominal pain, altered appetite, muscle weakness, bone pain. Extreme acidosis can cause weakness, confusion, convulsions, heartbeat abnormalities and low blood pressure. Lactic acidosis makes breath smell of acetone (nail-polish remover) or pear drops. People with coronary artery disease may have an abnormal heartbeat and angina (chest pain on exercise).

Treatment: Identify and treat the cause. For very severe acidosis (below pH 7.1), doctors may give intravenous (IV) sodium bicarbonate. If less severe (pH 7-7.35), they occasionally give IV or oral sodium bicarbonate. Oral bicarbonate can help soon after an aspirin overdose.

Respiratory acidosis

This is associated with excess retention of carbon dioxide in the blood, resulting from abnormally slow or interrupted breathing. The causes include:

- Certain medications, including anaesthetics and sedatives

- Brain injury, tumour or infection affecting the brain's breathing-control centre

- Playing a wind instrument, swimming underwater or other activity involving spasmodic breathing

- Pneumonia or other problems that reduce the exchange of oxygen and carbon dioxide in the lungs

- Severe asthma, chronic bronchitis, emphysema, pneumonia, airway obstruction, pneumothorax or other problems that increase airway resistance

- Obesity, burns, chest injury, polio, muscular dystrophy, Guillain-Barré syndrome, chest-wall deformity, scoliosis or other conditions that impede breathing by reducing chest-wall movement.

What happens? The kidneys try to compensate by excreting more hydrogen and less bicarbonate.

Symptoms: headache, drowsiness, fatigue, nausea, vomiting and exhaustion.

Treatment: Identify and treat the cause.

Metabolic alkalosis

This is associated with raised bicarbonate caused by the body losing too much acid or gaining too much alkali. The causes include:

- Loss of chloride due to repeated vomiting or repeated severe diarrhoea originating in the large intestine (for example, from ulcerative colitis, or the ongoing overuse of laxatives), or certain diuretics (medications that increase urine production)

- Low potassium from a poor diet, vomiting, overactive adrenal glands or diuretics. The kidneys retain sodium to take its place, but the resulting loss of hydrogen in urine makes blood over-alkaline

- Dehydration, diuretics, heart failure, bleeding, severe burns, or other causes of low blood and extracellular-fluid volume. The kidneys respond by retaining sodium, but the resulting hydrogen loss makes blood over-alkaline

- Steroid medication

- Too much IV bicarbonate medication

- Rarely, too much antacid medication.

What happens? Compensation by the body's pH-balancing mechanisms returns the pH to normal but leaves bicarbonate and carbon dioxide high.

Symptoms: Nausea and vomiting; numbness or tingling in the hands, feet and face; tremor; muscle twitching; cramp; dizziness; fainting; confusion.

Treatment: Identify and treat the cause. Water is replaced, if necessary with sodium and potassium, by IV infusion. Very severe alkalemia can be treated with IV dilute acid.

Respiratory alkalosis

This is associated with low carbon dioxide in the blood, caused by rapid breathing. The causes include:

- Anxiety

- Pain

- Fever

- Aspirin overdose (can also cause metabolic acidosis)

- Low oxygen from lung disease or high altitude.

What happens? The kidneys try to compensate, partly by excreting more bicarbonate.

Symptoms: Nausea and vomiting; numbness or tingling in the hands, feet and face; tremor; muscle twitching; cramp; dizziness; fainting; confusion.

Treatment: Identify and treat the cause. Slower breathing can help if anxiety or pain is responsible, as can breathing in and out of a large paper (not plastic) bag to raise the blood's carbon-dioxide level.

Does mild acidosis cause symptoms?

Researchers claim that almost all adults eating a typical Western diet have mild ongoing acidosis. The question is whether this 'chronic low-grade metabolic acidosis' can cause symptoms. Experts have long contested the idea, but we now know it can happen. For an excellent review, read, 'Diet-induced acidosis: is it real and clinically relevant?' in the *British Journal of Nutrition* (2010) 103, 1185–1194.

Whether such symptoms result from the lungs, kidneys and buffers compensating for the threat to the normal range of pH, or from a slight reduction in pH that nevertheless remains within the normal range, is unclear.

What causes mild acidosis?

It seems sensible to assume that any cause of metabolic acidosis with a pH below 7.35 could, if less severe, cause mild metabolic acidosis. But researchers think the two *main* causes of mild metabolic acidosis are:

- An acid-forming diet

- An age-related decline in kidney function.

We cannot prevent ageing, but we can adjust our diet (see Chapter 6). We can also deal with conditions that can cause more severe metabolic acidosis and might therefore cause the mild type. Finally, we can consider taking an alkali supplement (see Chapter 7).

Acid–alkali balance in the digestive tract

The efficiency of saliva, stomach juice, bile, pancreatic juice and intestinal juice depend on their pH.

Saliva

A high level of bicarbonate in saliva helps to neutralize acidic foods and enable the pytalin (an enzyme also called salivary amylase) to start breaking down starches into sugar. The pH of saliva between meals is 6.3 or above.

Stomach

Certain stomach-lining glands produce mucus that has a pH of 7.7 and contains large quantities (up to 0.5g a day) of sodium bicarbonate. This alkaline mucus protects the stomach from its own acid. Bicarbonate production rises if blood pH falls, and vice versa.

Other stomach-lining glands enable sodium and chloride ions to join with water and carbon dioxide to form hydrochloric acid (stomach acid) and sodium bicarbonate. For each molecule of acid produced, one of sodium bicarbonate is produced, too. All food stimulates stomach-acid production by distending the stomach, but protein is the main stimulus. Hydrochloric acid is released into the stomach, but bicarbonate ions are absorbed from the glands into the blood. Hydrochloric acid (stomach acid) has a pH of 1–3 and, along with the enzyme pepsinogen, alters proteins to make them more easily digestible. It also kills most of the micro-organisms we consume.

Alkaline tide: Blood leaving the stomach is relatively alkaline as it is rich in bicarbonate and short of chloride. As this 'alkaline tide' circulates around the body, its raised alkalinity helps to reduce any acidosis resulting from a meal.

The more acid-producing a meal (meaning the more acid it produces after digestion and metabolism), the more sodium bicarbonate is produced by the stomach and absorbed into the blood. That way the body fluids have enough to buffer a meal's acid-forming effects. However, the more sodium bicarbonate that is produced, the more stomach acid is produced, too. So an acid-forming meal increases stomach-acid production. Any excess acid is absorbed into the blood, which adds to its acid load. Conversely, when we have an alkali-producing meal, our stomach doesn't need to produce large amounts of sodium bicarbonate, so it doesn't produce large amounts of stomach acid either.

Several hours after a meal, the stomach contents enter the duodenum as an acidic 'sludge'.

Low stomach-acid production. This can result from ageing, stress, the prolonged use of antacid or acid-suppressant medication, or an acid-producing diet. It affects one in two people aged over 60.

It is possible, though unproven, that low stomach-acid production might also result from insufficient dietary potassium (mainly from vegetables and fruit). The body would then use sodium instead of potassium to accompany acids as they are excreted in urine. Sodium would be mobilized from various places, including stomach-acid-producing cells, and this would reduce stomach-acid production. Possible problems from too little stomach acid include:

- Malnutrition – because a lack of acid discourages the absorption of proteins, vitamins B and C, calcium, chromium, iron, magnesium, selenium and zinc

- Allergy – because too little acid means proteins aren't prepared for digestion; poorly digested proteins can then be absorbed from the intestine into the blood and cause allergic sensitization

- Gallstones – because too little acid discourages gallbladder contractions, and gallstones form more easily in stagnant bile

- Gastritis and peptic ulcer – because too little acid strongly correlates with *Helicobacter pylori* bacterial infection. An ulcer can develop if anything interferes with the stomach lining's cells or protective mucus. The usual culprit is inflammation (gastritis) from *H. pylori* infection. This also encourages stomach cancer.

Liver

Bicarbonate in bile helps to alkalinize stomach contents after their arrival in the duodenum. The liver also produces enzymes that alkalinize blood. Raised levels (indicated by liver-function blood tests) suggest that the liver is working overtime to help maintain a normal blood pH. The liver also influences the concentration of weak acids in body fluids.

Pancreas

Pancreatic juice is very alkaline because it receives a lot of sodium but not much chloride from the blood.

Secretin, a hormone produced by the duodenum, stimulates bicarbonate production in pancreatic-duct cells. The more acidic the food residues in the duodenum, the more secretin is produced.

Small intestine

Many factors influence the pH in the duodenum, including the size and timing of meals, the proportions of strong cations and anions (see page 63) from food, and the volume and pH of the stomach contents, bile and pancreatic juice. The resulting pH of about 7 activates pancreatic enzymes, including trypsinogen and chymotrypsinogen (which break down proteins into amino acids), lipase (which breaks down fats into fatty acids) and amylase (which breaks down starches to sugar).

Glands in the lining of the small intestine produce large amounts of alkaline fluid containing bicarbonate, which helps to neutralize any remaining stomach acid. Chloride from stomach acid, bicarbonate from pancreatic juice and strong ions from food are absorbed into the blood. All this takes hours, which suits the slow pace of the kidneys' pH-regulating mechanisms.

Colon

Water and strong ions, such as sodium and potassium, can be absorbed here. The colon is more alkaline than the small intestine because it has less chloride.

Glossary

Acid: a substance that can neutralize a base and increase the hydrogen-ion concentration of a watery solution.

Alkali: a base that increases the hydroxide-ion concentration of a watery solution.

Anion: a negatively charged ion.

Strong acidic anions: anions that can form acids (for example, hydrochloric, sulphuric and lactic) when combined with hydrogen ions.

Base: a substance that can neutralize an acid and decrease the hydrogen-ion concentration of a watery solution.

Cation: a positively charged ion.

Strong alkaline cations: strong cations that can form alkali when combined with weak anions.

Electrolyte: a substance that reversibly breaks down into ions in a watery solution. Strong electrolytes break down into ions completely in a watery solution. Weak electrolytes break down only partially.

Hydrogen atom: an electron (a particle with a negative electrical charge) plus a proton (a particle with a positive charge).

Hydrogen ion: a hydrogen atom minus its electron. This positively charged particle is 1800 times smaller than a hydrogen atom so has a particularly powerful electric field. This makes it react unusually rapidly with other ions, explaining its importance in acid-base balance.

Hydroxide ion: an ion made of one atom each of oxygen and hydrogen that between them have lost a proton, producing a negative electrical charge.

Ion: an atom or molecule that, when dissolved in water, has a positive or negative charge because it loses or gains one or more electrons. Strong ions come from strong electrolytes. Weak ions come from weak electrolytes.

CHAPTER 5

Balancing your diet

An acid-producing diet is the norm in the Western world. Such a diet lacks enough alkali-producing vegetables and fruit to balance the intake of acid-producing meat, fish, eggs and cereal-grain food, and the result is chronic low-grade metabolic acidosis. Bicarbonate plays an important part in the regulating systems that help our body counter acidosis.

Acidic foods

An acidic food is *not* the same as an acid-producing food. Acidic foods taste acidic because they contain organic food acids (such as citric, acetic, oxalic, malic, pyruvic and acetylsalicylic acids), 'organic' here meaning that they contain only carbon, oxygen and hydrogen. Some acidic foods, such as citrus fruit, vinegar, yoghurt, soured (sour) cream, buttermilk and soured milk, actually taste acidic. Others, such as beer, cider (apple cider), honey, treacle (molasses), maple syrup, coffee, and 'natural' cocoa and chocolate (dark unsweetened varieties made from cocoa beans that haven't been 'Dutch-processed') are acidic but don't taste so.

Organic food acids don't produce acid in the body because the liver breaks them down into carbon dioxide and water. Excess carbon dioxide is exhaled and excess water is eliminated by the kidneys and lungs. So most acidic foods have virtually no effect on our acid–alkali balance; a few, including lemon juice and cider vinegar (apple cider vinegar), even have an alkali-producing effect.

Acid-producing foods

These foods are not acidic and do not taste acidic, but when digested and metabolized produce acids that make body fluids less alkaline. An acid-producing diet is rich in meat, grain and sugar and carbonated drinks and low in vegetables and fruit.

Certain acid-producing foods produce acid by releasing more strong acidic anions (such as sulphate/sulfate, which can join with hydrogen ions to form sulphuric acid) than strong alkaline cations (see page 63), such as potassium, which can join with bicarbonate to form potassium bicarbonate.

The kidneys can eliminate only a limited load of strong acidic ions each hour, so any surplus causes acidosis.

Acid-producing foods include:

- Protein (such as in meat, fish, eggs, cheese, beans)

- Grain foods (such as bread, breakfast cereal, pasta, cakes, biscuits, many puddings, and rice; note that refined-grain foods are more acid-producing than wholegrain foods)

- Sugar (especially refined sugar – both white and brown).

Certain acid-producing foods and food constituents have an acidifying effect that is independent of the diet's total acid-producing load:

- Table salt (sodium chloride) encourages acidosis by decreasing the blood's strong-ion difference. (It does this by increasing chloride more than sodium and encouraging the kidneys to excrete potassium.)

- Tea, coffee, cocoa, chocolate and pulses and legumes (such as soya beans and chickpeas) contain purines that are metabolized to uric acid.

- Alcohol encourages acidosis by increasing lactate production.

Foods that cause an 'acid tummy'

Strongly acidic foods (such as lemon juice), plus certain acid-producing foods and drinks, can stimulate the production of enough stomach acid to cause 'acid indigestion'. Such foods include those made from white sugar or white flour; tea, coffee (even decaffeinated) and cocoa; and beer and wine (possibly because of protein-breakdown products such as amino acids and amines produced during fermentation).

Alkali-producing foods

These foods contain more strong alkaline than strong acidic ions, so when metabolized, they produce alkaline salts such as bicarbonate. They include:

- vegetables and fruit

- certain nuts, beans, grains, cheeses and sugars.

Many experts assert that alkali-producing foods should compose 80 per cent of our diet, with acid-producing foods making up the rest. However, the average Western diet is composed mainly of acid-producing foods, with vegetables and fruit (the major alkali-producing foods) contributing only 2 per cent!

Our diet

The effect of our overall diet on our acid–alkali balance is more important than the effects of individual foods. This is because, when a meal has been digested and metabolized, its net effect is either acidic or alkaline.

Our aim should be to eat an alkali-producing diet. We can deal with temporary acidosis from an occasional acid-producing meal, but weeks or months of chronic low-grade acidosis may cause symptoms.

Research published in the *American Journal of Clinical Nutrition* (1998; 68:576–583) suggests the two key factors affecting our acid–alkali balance are our intake of:

- protein (especially meat), which is acidifying, and

- potassium (most importantly, from vegetables and fruits), which is alkalinizing.

The US Third National Health and Nutrition Examination Survey of 33,994 people in 1988–94 found that the average American diet is acid-producing. However, studies suggest that in the pre-agricultural societies of over 70,000 years ago, 87 per cent of people ate an alkali-producing diet. So it is likely that a huge change in eating patterns has occurred over the millennia.

Protein
Animal protein is found in meat, fish, eggs and dairy food. Research suggests that dairy food's high calcium levels help to protect against any acidosis-promoting effect of its protein. Vegetable protein is found mainly in beans and peas and in nuts, grains and other seeds.

Potassium
Potassium is plentiful in vegetables and fruits and produces strong alkalizing ions in body fluids. Particularly rich sources include green leafy vegetables, tomatoes, bananas, dates and avocados.

What are acid-producing and alkali-producing foods and drinks?

Burning a food in a laboratory produces heat and reduces the food to acidic or alkaline ash. This is the equivalent of our cells burning food to produce energy. So measuring the pH of a burnt food's ash indicates the acid- or alkali-producing effect of that food in our body. The ash produced by the average vegetarian diet is significantly more alkaline that that from the average omnivorous diet. This is mainly because animal protein has a particularly high acid-producing potential.

THE ACID-PRODUCING POTENTIAL OF VARIOUS FOODS

'High', 'Medium' and 'Low' refer to a food's acid-producing potential. Most of us could do with eating less 'high' acid-producing food:

Meat and fish	High:	Pork, beef, shellfish
	Medium:	Eggs, lamb, sea fish, chicken
	Low:	Freshwater fish
Dairy foods	High:	Hard cheese, ice cream
	Medium:	Soft cheese, cream
	Low:	Yoghurt, cottage cheese, milk
Grain-foods	High:	White flour, white bread, white pasta
	Medium:	Wholemeal and wholegrain bread; biscuits, white rice, corn, oats
	Low:	Brown rice, sprouted-wheat (Essene) bread, spelt flour and bread
Nuts	Medium:	Pistachios, peanuts, cashews, walnuts
	Low:	Macadamias, hazelnuts
Fats and oils	Low:	Margarine, sunflower oil, corn oil, butter
Sugar, honey, confectionery	Medium:	Chocolate, white sugar, brown sugar
	Low:	Processed honey, treacle (molasses)

| **Condiments** | High: | Most vinegar, soy sauce, salt |
| | Medium: | Mustard, mayonnaise, tomato ketchup. |

Drinks	High:	Spirits, beer, soft drinks
	Medium:	Coffee, wine, fruit juice
	Low:	Tea

| **Vegetables** | Medium: | Potatoes without skins; pinto, navy and lima beans |
| | Low: | Kidney beans |

| **Fruits** | Medium: | Cranberries |
| | Low: | Plums, prunes |

| **Other** | Low: | Coconut milk |

THE ALKALI-PRODUCING POTENTIAL OF VARIOUS FOODS

'High', 'Medium' and 'Low' refer to a food's alkali-producing potential. Most of us could do with eating or drinking more of these foods:

Fruits	Medium:	Avocado, tomato, lemon, dried figs, rhubarb
	Low:	Pineapple, raisins, dried dates, strawberries, grapefruit, apricot, blackberries, orange, peach, raspberries, banana, grapes, pear, blueberries, apple, coconut
Vegetables	High:	Cucumber, sprouted seeds
	Medium:	Radishes, celery, garlic, spinach, beetroot (beet), French beans, carrots, chives, turnips
	Low:	Watercress, leeks, courgettes (zucchini), peas, cabbage, cauliflower, mushrooms, swede (rutabaga), onion, lettuce, potatoes with skins, asparagus, Brussels sprouts, sweet potatoes
Beans	Medium:	White ('navy') beans, fresh (or frozen) soya beans (soybeans)
	Low:	Tofu, soya flour, lentils
Dairy food	Low:	Goat's cheese, goat's milk, soya milk, buttermilk
Grains	Low:	Buckwheat, spelt, wild rice, quinoa
Nuts and seeds	Low:	Almonds, Brazil nuts, chestnuts, pumpkin seeds, sunflower seeds, flaxseeds, sesame seeds

Oils	Medium:	Olive oil, flaxseed oil
	Low:	Rapeseed oil (canola), olive oil
Sugar, honey	High:	Raw honey, raw sugar
	Medium:	Maple syrup
Drinks	High:	Herb tea, lemon water
	Medium:	Green tea
	Low:	Ginger tea
Other	Low:	Cider vinegar (apple cider vinegar)

How to improve your diet

If you have been eating a typical Western diet, help to rebalance it by using the above lists as a guide to favouring alkali-producing foods. An added bonus is that the vegetable and fruit content of such a diet provides a wealth of health-enhancing factors, including vitamins, phenolic compounds, carotenoids, plant hormones, salicylates, fibre and omega-3 fats.

- As already noted, research shows that the two factors that best predict acidosis are too much protein (especially too much red meat) and not enough potassium (mainly from vegetables and fruit). However, although the matter is still being studied, my understanding is that a lack of vegetables and fruit is the most likely cause of health problems from a typical Western diet.

- Eat at least five servings a day of vegetables and fruit, of which three should be vegetables, two fruit. Potatoes (and yams, cassava and plantain) are important for an alkali-producing diet as they are potassium-rich. However, they don't count towards your five-a-day as they are classed not as vegetables but as starchy carbohydrates (like bread, rice, noodles, pasta and sweetcorn). Peas, beans and lentils count as only one helping a day, no matter how much you eat, because they contain fewer nutrients than do other vegetables. However, sweet potatoes, parsnips, swedes and turnips *do* count towards your five-a-day. Fruit and vegetable juices count as only one helping a day, however much you drink.

- Five-a-day is officially recommended in the US and many other countries. But one large US study (*American Journal of Preventive Medicine*, 2007) found that only 32 per cent of people met the guidelines for vegetables, only 28 per cent for fruits, and fewer than 11 per cent for vegetables *and* fruit. Also, one in four ate no vegetables on a daily basis and three in five ate no whole fruits!

- Some experts recommend up to nine helpings of vegetables a day, as well as two of fruit. This would certainly decrease your appetite for acid-producing foods!

  Cook vegetables lightly and use the potassium-rich cooking water in soups or gravy, or eat them raw.

- Include alkali-producing food in every meal and snack.

- Keep a food diary of everything you consume over seven days. Highlight acid-producing foods in red, alkali-producing in green. This will help you to evaluate the balance of your diet.

- Use the Diet Plate, or the Eatwell Plate, developed by the food standards agency in the UK (see page 130).

- Avoid added salt, use less, or choose potassium-enriched 'low' salt.

CHAPTER 6

Ailments and natural remedies

You can treat yourself with sodium bicarbonate in three different ways. The first is by changing to an alkali-producing diet, of which full details are given in Chapter 5. Changing to an alkali-producing diet is the most important starting point for nearly all the common ailments in this chapter. Two other methods are taking sodium bicarbonate by mouth, or applying it to the skin as a paste or in a bath.

Take sodium bicarbonate

Sodium bicarbonate is available from supermarkets and groceries as 'bicarbonate of soda' in the UK and 'baking soda' in the US. It is not the same as 'baking powder' (see page 25).

Dose

One teaspoon of the powder contains 600mg of sodium bicarbonate. The usual adult dose, taken 1–4 times a day, is:

Under-60s: ½–1 teaspoon   Over-60s: ¼–½ teaspoon

In the UK, sodium bicarbonate is also available from pharmacies as 500mg capsules and 600mg tablets. In the US, it is available as 325mg and 650mg tablets.

The US Food and Drug Administration (FDA) sets the maximum dose at 16g per day for the under-60s; 8g per day for the over-60s.

For optimal absorption into the blood, take sodium bicarbonate on an empty stomach. For acid indigestion, take it when you have discomfort. Doctors sometimes give sodium bicarbonate in an intravenous (IV) 'drip'.

As sodium bicarbonate neutralizes stomach acid, it releases carbon dioxide, which causes belching. Any excess sodium bicarbonate passes into the intestine and, when absorbed into the blood, has an alkalinizing effect.

Tips and warnings

- Don't take sodium bicarbonate daily for more than 2 weeks without consulting a doctor.

- Don't confuse it with baking powder.

- Unless agreed with your doctor, don't take it if you're on a sodium-restricted diet or have high blood pressure, kidney, lung, heart or liver disease, fluid retention, urination problems, low blood calcium or anal bleeding.

- Take only small doses if pregnant, breastfeeding or over 60.

- Consult your doctor first if you are on prescription drugs, as some interact with sodium bicarbonate. Some of those that do interact include benzodiazepines, calcium- or citrate-containing preparations, ephedrine, fluoroquinolones, iron, ketoconazole, lithium, methenamine, oral anti-diabetes drugs, quinidine, steroids, tetracycline and urine-acidifying medications.

- Check with a doctor or sports coach if considering taking sodium bicarbonate to enhance your exercise performance.

- Don't give sodium bicarbonate to a child unless discussed with a doctor and the dose agreed.

Side effects

Depending on the dose and the person, sodium bicarbonate can cause:

- Metabolic alkalosis, with nausea, vomiting, numbness, tingling, tremor, muscle twitching, cramp, dizziness, fainting, confusion

- High blood sodium, possibly with thirst, ankle swelling, high blood pressure, frequent urination, seizures, heart failure or even a stroke

- Low blood potassium, possibly with weakness, fatigue, cramp, tingling, numbness, nausea, vomiting, bloating, constipation, irregular heartbeat, large amounts of urine, thirst, confusion, hallucinations or fainting

- Nervous-system depression, possibly with headache, drowsiness, nausea, vomiting, lack of coordination, dizziness or confusion

- Milk-alkali syndrome – abnormally high blood calcium in people with poor kidney function, if sodium bicarbonate is taken with dairy products, calcium supplements or calcium-containing antacids. If continued, this can cause calcium deposits, kidney stones and kidney failure

- Allergic swelling of the face, lips, tongue and throat, and difficulty in breathing. This needs urgent medical attention.

If you suspect a serious reaction, or have taken an overdose, call a doctor or an ambulance; in the US, call the National Poison Control Center on 1-800-222-1222. If you go to a doctor or hospital, you or someone else should bring the container of sodium bicarbonate.

How to make soda water

Drinking soda water is a pleasant way of taking sodium bicarbonate.

Make it with a 1-litre/35fl oz/4 cup rechargeable soda siphon, a disposable one-shot screw-in cartridge of pressurized carbon dioxide, plus sodium bicarbonate and water.

Add ¼–½ teaspoon of sodium bicarbonate to 1 litre/35fl oz/4 cups of water. Put this into the soda siphon, then add the carbon dioxide.

Flavour it with plain syrup or fruit syrup if you like.

Unlike many soft drinks, soda water does not contain phosphoric acid, which encourages calcium loss from bones.

Alternatives to sodium bicarbonate

If you cannot take sodium bicarbonate for some reason, discuss with your doctor whether an alternative alkalinizer (such as potassium bicarbonate or calcium carbonate) would be appropriate.

Apply sodium bicarbonate to the skin

Sodium bicarbonate dissolved in water has an alkaline pH of 8.3 and can ease the itching, discomfort and inflammation of certain skin conditions. Two ways of applying it are making it into a paste or adding it to a bath.

Sodium-bicarbonate paste

Put 1 tablespoon of sodium bicarbonate into a small bowl and stir in about 1 teaspoon of water. Apply a thin layer of the paste to the skin. Let the paste dry on the skin, then leave it on for 30 minutes before rinsing it off with water.

Alkaline bath

Add 100–200g/3½–7oz/½–1 cup of sodium bicarbonate to a bath of comfortably hot water. Add a few drops of lavender or other essential oil for fragrance.

Testing urine pH

Unusually acidic urine suggests that the kidneys are eliminating excess acid. The most common reason for this is an acid-forming diet.

The pH of normal urine ranges from 4.6 to 8.0. It's more acidic in the morning than in the evening. If you test your urine, it's best to test '24-hour' urine (all the urine passed in 24 hours and pooled in one container, or cupfuls collected each time you urinate and pooled in one container). Urine pH test strips are available from pharmacies or on the internet.

Ailments

Please note:

- Every ailment has many possible causes. Only those pertaining to sodium bicarbonate or the body's acid–alkali balance are included here.

- Consult a doctor about possible causes and treatments for continuing, worrying or worsening symptoms.

- You can help prevent and treat most ailments with a healthy diet, adequate hydration, regular exercise, daily outdoor light, effective stress management, a sensible alcohol intake and no smoking.

- When I mention a study, I give the journal's name and year of publication. These, plus some keywords, should enable you to find out more on the internet.

Anxiety

Anxiety can encourage either acidosis or alkalosis. In addition, acidosis can encourage anxiety. One way in which anxiety can cause acidosis is by increasing the stress hormone adrenaline. This tenses muscles, which in turn boosts energy production in muscle-cells, releasing an acidic anion called lactate.

Urine from people having a panic attack is unusually acidic.
(*Psychiatry Research*, 2005)

Increased adrenaline production can cause acidosis.
(*Clinical Science*, 1983)

Conversely, some anxious people breathe rapidly, so they exhale too much carbon dioxide, encouraging respiratory alkalosis (see page 70).

As for acidosis encouraging anxiety, people on a high-protein diet have acidosis and are allegedly more likely to feel irritable. Also, chronic acidosis encourages anxiety by encouraging magnesium loss from bones.

Action: Eat an alkali-forming diet (see page 84–5).

Arthritis

Rheumatoid arthritis is linked with the intake of meat, wheat, sugar, salt and coffee – all of which are acid-producing:

> Daily meat consumption was associated with double the risk compared with eating it less often. More protein in general was implicated too.
>
> *(Arthritis and Rheumatism, 2004)*

> A study at the University of Oslo associated meat, wine and coffee with joint swelling.
>
> *(Plant Foods for Human Nutrition, 1993)*

Other research indicates a lower likelihood in Mediterranean countries, where the traditional diet contains little red meat. Rheumatoid arthritis is also less common in vegetarians and vegans who, in turn, are less likely than meat-eaters to have an acid-forming diet. And it's less common in people who eat more cruciferous vegetables (such as cabbage and broccoli) and fruit:

> A US study found rheumatoid arthritis was less likely in women who ate more fruit and cruciferous vegetables.
>
> *(American Journal of Epidemiology, 2003)*

People with rheumatoid arthritis are more likely to have antibodies to milk, cereal, eggs, fish and pork. Food sensitivity is encouraged by an acid-producing diet. So it's possible that such a diet might encourage rheumatoid symptoms as part of an immune response triggered by a food sensitivity (see 'Food allergy', pages 104–5). All this suggests that an acid-forming diet encourages rheumatoid arthritis.

Osteoarthritis can be linked with acidosis. The kidneys normally excrete acidic salts, but if they can't do this fast enough, such salts can crystallize in joint fluid and trigger inflammation:

Research at the University of Padova in Italy shows that joint fluid in people with osteoarthritis may contain crystals, including those of calcium pyrophosphate dihydrate (present in one in three), apatite (present in one in four) and silicon dioxide.

(*Journal of Rheumatology*, 2008)

Irish researchers discovered that deposits in joints of crystals of octacalcium phosphate, tricalcium phosphate, carbonate-substituted hydroxyapatite and magnesium whitlockite can be to blame for both osteoarthritis and the inflammatory joint condition *calcific periarthritis*.

(*Current Rheumatology Reports*, 2003)

Gout causes arthritis and can be triggered by acidosis (see page 106).

Action: Eat an alkali-producing diet.

Asthma

Food allergy triggered by an acid-producing diet can be responsible for asthma (see 'Food allergy', pages 104–5). Pre-existing acidosis also makes airway-widening medication less effective early in an attack.

Airway tightening during an attack triggers deep rapid breathing. Too much carbon dioxide is then exhaled, leading to respiratory alkalosis. This triggers the bicarbonate buffering system to normalize the alkalosis. But if a person's diet is acid-producing, they could be short of bicarbonate, in which case their alkalosis might continue or even worsen.

Breathing exercises can help:

> An Australian study found that shallow nose breathing ('Buteyko breathing'), or steady nose or mouth breathing (plus upper-body exercises, relaxation and good posture), during an attack decreased reliever-inhaler use by 86 percent, and halved the dose of inhaled-steroid medication.
>
> (*Thorax*, 2006)

Sodium bicarbonate can relax airways and encourage them to respond to airway-widening medication.

> Intravenous sodium bicarbonate improves blood pH and carbon-dioxide concentration in children with life-threatening asthma.
>
> (*Chest*, 2005)

Action: Eat an alkali-producing diet.

Consider taking sodium bicarbonate.

Bad breath

An acid-forming diet encourages bad breath from residues of meat or refined carbohydrate on or between the teeth. Mouth bacteria can break these down and release unpleasant-smelling compounds.

The cells of people who eat a high-protein, low-carbohydrate diet, or have uncontrolled diabetes, must produce energy from fats instead of sugar. This leads to a build-up of acidic ketones in the blood. These taint breath with the scent of peardrops or nail-polish remover.

> A study at Duke University found that 63 percent of people on a high-protein, low-carbohydrate diet reported bad breath.
>
> (*American Journal of Medicine*, 2002)

Action: Rinse your mouth with ½ teaspoon of sodium bicarbonate in a glass of water.

Eat a well-balanced, alkali-forming diet.

Seek urgent medical help if your breath smells of ketones and you have diabetes or suspect you might have it.

Cancer

Early research increasingly supports the idea that acidosis can encourage cancer. For example, studies indicate that cancer cells sometimes stop multiplying when the pH is relatively alkaline (just above 7.4). This pH also encourages more oxygen to enter cancer cells – which is good because low oxygen encourages cancer cells to multiply. Other research shows that cancer cells engender acidosis around them, which makes weak-alkali anti-cancer drugs less effective.

Several links suggest that acidosis encourages cancer:

- Obesity is associated with more bowel, gallbladder, kidney and prostate cancers. Researchers also speculate that acidosis encourages obesity. So acidosis may prove to be an underlying factor behind both obesity and cancer.

- A high protein intake encourages bowel and prostate cancer, whereas eating plenty of vegetables discourages bowel, breast and stomach cancer. Similarly, an acid-producing diet encourages acidosis. So acidosis may prove to encourage certain cancers.

- Studies suggest that acidosis encourages diabetes. People with diabetes have an increased risk of certain cancers (for example, liver and pancreas cancer). So acidosis may prove to encourage both diabetes and cancer.

Researchers report that:

> Giving sodium bicarbonate to mice with cancer alkalinizes the area around the cancer.
>
> *(British Journal of Radiology*, 2003)

If the above also applies to humans, it would enable weak-alkali anti-cancer drugs to work. What's more:

> Oral sodium bicarbonate increases cancer pH, reduces cancer growth, inhibits metastases (secondary cancers) and discourages lymph-node involvement in mice with cancer.
>
> *(Cancer Research*, 2009)

Unproven treatment claims include:

- Applying sodium-bicarbonate paste to a rodent ulcer (basal-cell carcinoma) or squamous-cell skin cancer.

- Taking ascorbic acid and sodium bicarbonate for stomach or bowel cancer. These release sodium ascorbate and the hope is that this will damage cancer cells.

- Taking sodium bicarbonate mixed with maple syrup.

Finally, bicarbonate is proving useful in diagnosing cancer and monitoring treatment. This is because cancer cells convert bicarbonate to carbon dioxide, and magnetic resonance imaging (MRI) scans can monitor changing carbon-dioxide levels.

Action: Eat an alkali-producing diet.

Cataracts

These could be linked with acidosis as they can result from ageing or stress encouraging a build-up in the eyes' lenses of insoluble calcium salts of phosphoric or uric acid. Taking sodium bicarbonate helps to dissolve these salts, as does a potassium-rich diet.

Action: Eat an alkali-producing diet, as this is rich in potassium and its metabolism produces bicarbonate.

Colic in babies

Many parents use gripe water to soothe their baby's 'colic' (restlessness, crying and hiccups attributed to intestinal spasm). All brands contain sugar plus small doses of ingredients such as sodium bicarbonate, fennel and ginger.

Gripe water isn't approved by the US Food and Drug Administration because imported brands may contain alcohol and sodium bicarbonate in amounts considered unsafe.

Action: If giving gripe water, check it contains no alcohol, follow the directions, and consult a doctor first if your baby is on other medication.

Confusion

This can be a symptom of severe metabolic acidosis – caused, for example, by serious heart, lung or liver disease.

Action: Seek urgent medical help.

Convulsions

Convulsions occur in 70–80 per cent of people with epilepsy, despite their medication, and acidosis may be a factor.

> Researchers believe the chronic low-grade metabolic acidosis associated with most modern Western diets encourages chronic epilepsy by over-exciting brain cells.
>
> *(Epilepsy and Behavior, 2006)*

Convulsions can also result from a slow-onset immune reaction caused by a food sensitivity enabled by acidosis (see 'Food allergy', pages 104–5).

Action: Eat an alkali-forming diet.

Cystitis

A person with acidosis produces relatively acidic urine. This can inflame the bladder and encourage urine infections. The resulting cystitis causes painful, frequent urination.

Alkalinizing the body with sodium bicarbonate helps to neutralize excess acid in the urine. It also kills bacteria and makes certain antibiotics more effective.

Action: Affected women should consider drinking ½ teaspoon of sodium bicarbonate in a glass of water four times a day. Other alkalinizing remedies are available from pharmacies.

See a doctor if this is your first attack, or you are no better within 2–3 days. Men and children should always see a doctor.

Depression

Depression is sometimes reported as a side-effect of a high-protein, low-carbohydrate diet, which in turn is associated with low-grade metabolic acidosis.

Depression can also result from a slow-onset immune reaction caused by a food sensitivity enabled by acidosis (see 'Food allergy', pages 104–5).

Action: Eat an alkali-producing diet.

Diabetes, pre-diabetes and metabolic syndrome

Researchers believe that acidosis encourages cells to become resistant to insulin. Normally, this hormone enables blood sugar to enter cells. But if cells are resistant, blood-sugar rises. The pancreas then produces extra insulin to prevent high blood sugar. This 'pre-diabetes' can have adverse effects, including obesity, fluid retention, high blood pressure, raised LDL-cholesterol, fatigue, faintness, mood swings, dry skin, skin tags and darkened skin.

Some people with pre-diabetes have a collection of problems together called the metabolic syndrome. This greatly encourages diabetes, heart disease and strokes and is characterized by having three of the following: insulin resistance, excess fat around the waist, high blood pressure, high blood fats, or low HDL-cholesterol (the helpful sort).

A study at the University of Texas reveals that overly acidic urine (which indicates acidosis) is a feature of the metabolic

syndrome and associated with the degree of insulin resistance.
(*Clinical Journal of the American Society of Nephrology*, 2007)

Continued insulin resistance can exhaust pancreatic cells, resulting in type 2 diabetes. People with diabetes tend to have overly acidic urine, indicating acidosis.

> Researchers at the University of Texas say that excess weight and an acid-producing diet can't entirely account for the overly acidic urine in people with diabetes.
> (*Journal of the American Society of Nephrology*, 2006)

Dieters may develop acidosis if their diet contains insufficient vegetables and fruit. This is a particular problem because many people with pre-diabetes, metabolic syndrome or diabetes are overweight and repeatedly trying to slim.

Before oral anti-diabetic drugs, and insulin, doctors often treated diabetes with sodium bicarbonate.

Action: In addition to whatever other treatment you need, eat an alkali-producing diet.

Diarrhoea

If persistent severe diarrhoea originates in the small intestine, it can cause metabolic acidosis from the loss of bicarbonate. If it originates in the large intestine it can cause metabolic alkalosis from the loss of chloride.

Diarrhoea can also result from a slow-onset immune reaction enabled by acidosis (see 'Food allergy', pages 104–5).

Action: Eat an alkali-producing diet.

Consider taking oral rehydration salts (from a pharmacy) or ½ teaspoon of sodium bicarbonate in a glass of water up to four times a day.

Dizziness, light-headedness and fainting

These can be associated with either respiratory or metabolic alkalosis (see pages 70–71 and 69–70).

They can also result from the acidosis that can accompany pre-diabetes and a slimming diet (particularly one low in carbohydrate).

Action: Check out these and other possible causes and treat as appropriate. Also, eat an alkali-producing diet.

Drowsiness

This could be a sign of respiratory or metabolic acidosis.

Action: For causes and treatments, see pages 69 and 70.

Fatigue and poor concentration

These can result from metabolic acidosis. One possible reason is exhaustion from rapid breathing triggered as the body tries to correct a low pH.

A second possible cause is a slimming diet, particularly if low in carbohydrate. This leads to a shortage of sugar for energy production and means cells must use protein or fat as an energy source instead. But converting these nutrients to usable fuels takes longer than converting carbohydrate to sugar. This is a particular disadvantage for brain cells, hence the fatigue and poor concentration. What's more, burning fat for energy produces acidic ketones. Not only can the resulting acidosis cause fatigue but it also encourages pre-diabetes, which can trigger tiredness. The lack of sugar also affects heart muscle (see 'Heart disease', page 107–8), causing low energy.

A third possible reason is a slow-onset immune reaction associated with a food sensitivity enabled by acidosis (see 'Food allergy', pages 104–5).

Action: Eat an alkali-producing diet.

Fibromyalgia

With this condition you have stiff, weak, knotted shoulder and back muscles and tender points on hips, knees, neck, spine, elbows or buttocks. There may also be fatigue, poor sleep, headaches, dizziness, numbness, tingling, irritable bowel and bladder, restless legs, poor memory and concentration, depression, anxiety, over-sensitivity to noise, light and temperature, and Raynaud's phenomenon.

Many experts blame metabolic acidosis, suggesting that this deposits acidic ions in muscles and connective tissue. Various studies support this idea, including:

A study at the University of Oslo in which most of the volunteers with fibromyalgia who ate a vegetarian diet for 3 weeks reported less pain and better well-being.

(*Plant Foods for Human Nutrition*, 1993)

Action: Eat an alkali-producing diet.

Food allergy

Chronic low-grade metabolic acidosis is associated with low bicarbonate in the body. This means pancreatic juice may not contain enough bicarbonate to alkalinize acidic food residues entering the duodenum. As a result, its enzymes may not break down proteins properly; also, acidic food residues can damage the intestinal lining. Whole undigested protein molecules can then pass through the 'leaky' lining into the blood and sensitize the immune system.

When someone sensitized to a protein next eats it, one of two things can happen. The first is that immunoglobuin E (IgE) antibodies can adhere to it in the intestine, blood or elsewhere, forming tiny particles called immune complexes, which can cause trouble (for example, by blocking tiny blood vessels). The second is that white cells can release inflammatory substances (such as histamine and leucotrienes), which can increase the production of potentially damaging free radicals (reactive oxygen-containing ions).

Food-allergic symptoms beginning within minutes or up to 2 hours are caused by a fast-action immune response. This can result from eating even only a little of the particular food. Common culprits are milk, eggs, peanuts, tree nuts, fish, shellfish, soya, wheat and oranges. Possible symptoms include swollen face, lips, mouth, tongue and throat; vomiting; diarrhoea; abdominal pain; itching; allergic rhinitis ('hayfever'); urticaria (hives or 'nettle-rash'); asthma; and conjunctivitis. Pre-existing eczema may worsen. At worst there is anaphylactic shock (with potentially fatal breathing difficulty, a fall in blood pressure and, perhaps, loss of consciousness).

Food-allergic symptoms beginning later, though within 72 hours, are caused by a slow-onset immune response. Affected people may react to several foods. Possible symptoms include flushing, nausea, vomiting, diarrhoea, oesophagitis (inflamed gullet), gastritis (inflamed stomach), abdominal pain, fatigue, muscle weakness, aching and stiffness, eczema, joint pains, palpitation, fluid retention (perhaps with bloating, headaches, fluctuating weight, temporarily raised blood pressure, depression, convulsions and restless legs) and gallstones.

Action: Eat an alkali-forming diet.

Consider taking sodium bicarbonate during an attack (though not if there are symptoms of fluid retention).

Gallbladder disease

The risk of gallstones or an inflamed gallbladder rises in people who lose weight rapidly, as this can cause acidosis. The risk of gallstones also rises in people who are obese, and certain experts believe that acidosis encourages obesity. None of this proves that acidosis causes gallstones, but it does suggest that it's possible.

On a different tack, acidosis encourages an immune response to certain proteins. People with gallstones have a raised risk of food sensitivity (see 'Food allergy', pages 104–5), the most likely culprits being eggs, pork, onions, chicken, milk and coffee. So acidosis might indirectly encourage gallstones. One suggested mechanism is that a food-sensitive immune response inflames the bile duct, making bile stagnate in the gallbladder and thus encouraging stones.

Action: Eat an alkali-producing diet.

Gout

Gout is associated with needle-like crystals of sodium urate (specifically, monosodium urate monohydrate) in joints or under the skin. Urates form when purines from food and from the body's cells are broken down by the body into uric acid, which is carried in the blood as urate. The kidneys normally excrete excess urate, but with acidosis they may not do so fast enough, so urate levels rise.

Some people report that taking sodium bicarbonate alleviates or cures an attack. By reducing acidosis, this presumably (it is not yet proven) enables more sodium urate to dissolve in the blood, encouraging urate crystals in the joints to dissolve. Gout attacks are more likely at night, which is when the body is particularly acidic.

In an online poll of people with gout, 85 per cent said that sodium bicarbonate helped.

Action: Consider taking ½ teaspoon of sodium bicarbonate four times a day for a week.

Eat an alkali-forming diet.

Headache

Headaches are a possible symptom of metabolic acidosis with a pH below 7.35. It's also possible, though unproven, that chronic low-grade metabolic acidosis can cause headaches as a result of the body's buffer systems working extra hard to keep the blood's acid–alkali balance within its normal tightly controlled range.

Another cause of headaches is a slow-onset immune reaction associated with a food sensitivity enabled by acidosis (see 'Food allergy', pages 104–5).

Action: If you eat an acid-producing diet or have other reason to believe you might have acidosis, consider taking ½–1 teaspoon of sodium bicarbonate in a glass of water to help cure a headache.

Eat an alkali-producing diet.

Heart disease

The findings below indicate that acidosis encourages low energy, an irregular heartbeat (atrial fibrillation), chest pain on exercise (angina), heart attacks and heart failure. Whether chronic low-grade metabolic acidosis (as with a typical Western diet) has similar effects isn't yet known.

Many studies show that acidosis can:

- Reduce energy production from sugar in heart-muscle cells; energy production from fats and proteins takes longer than from sugar, so low energy is an early problem.

- Irritate the coronary arteries (if the pH is below 7.35),
encouraging tiny tears. LDL-cholesterol then seeps into the
artery lining and attracts white blood cells. These white cells
provoke inflammation, which oxidizes cholesterol. They then
engulf the oxidized cholesterol. Calcium infiltrates the damaged
artery walls, while smooth-muscle cells produce collagen to
cover the leaks. All this causes atherosclerosis – stiffening of the
arteries plus narrowing by a chalky, fatty, fibrous, white-cell-
laden substance called atheroma building up in the artery walls.
Patches of atheroma can rupture, encouraging a blood clot,
which could trigger a heart attack.

- Interfere with the passage of potassium, sodium and calcium
across cell membranes, and also rob the body of potassium,
calcium and magnesium as they neutralize acids in the urine.
This weakens heart-muscle, prevents the normal conduction of
electrical messages, and makes sodium and calcium accumulate
in blood, encouraging high blood pressure and atheroma.

- Increase LDL-cholesterol (the sort that's potentially dangerous if
oxidized) and decrease HDL-cholesterol (the protective sort).

- Increase adrenaline, which speeds the heart and boosts its cells'
need for oxygen.

- Encourage insulin-resistance; blood sugar then can't enter cells
normally, so rises, triggering extra insulin production. But high
insulin has adverse effects, such as boosting LDL-cholesterol.

- Raise fibrinogen, encouraging blood clots, which can block a
coronary artery.

For example:

> Acidosis rapidly reduces the passage of calcium into heart-muscle cells. This prevents the heart pumping efficiently and rhythmically. The greater the acidosis, the less well the heart pumps.
>
> *(Ciba Foundation Symposium*, 1982)

Blood pH is lowest (at its most acidotic) during sleep, which is when fatal heart attacks are most common.

Palpitation can result from a slow-onset immune reaction associated with a food sensitivity enabled by acidosis (see 'Food allergy', pages 104–5).

Action: Eat an alkali-producing diet.

High blood pressure

Acidosis seems to encourage high blood pressure:

> In a study of 15,385 women, those whose diets had a higher potential acid load had higher blood pressure than those with a lower load.
>
> *(Hypertension*, 2009)

The probable culprit is a lack of vegetables and fruit, since there is no evidence that a high protein intake in itself raises blood pressure.

Taking sodium bicarbonate (or any other alkalizer) may reduce blood pressure:

> Consuming sodium bicarbonate as part of a low-salt diet can lower blood pressure by reducing calcium excretion in urine.
>
> *(Journal of Hypertension*, January 1996, Vol. 14, Issue 1)

Acidosis makes cells more resistant to insulin. The pancreas then produces extra insulin to prevent high blood sugar. This makes arteries over-sensitive to adrenaline, thereby encouraging high blood pressure.

Action: Eat an alkali-producing diet.

Indigestion, heartburn, gastritis and peptic ulcer

Acidosis from an acid-producing diet increases the stomach's production of bicarbonate *and* acid. The acid encourages 'acid' indigestion, heartburn, peptic ulcers and gastritis (inflamed stomach lining). When the stomach contents enter the duodenum, pancreatic juice provides bicarbonate to neutralize the acid. This stimulates stomach-lining cells to produce more bicarbonate; at the same time they automatically produce even more acid.

Taking sodium bicarbonate can neutralize excess acid. But its sodium is absorbed into the blood and some people are believed to be sodium-sensitive. So antacids such as calcium carbonate or magnesium or aluminium hydroxide are probably preferable (and scarcely absorbed). Antacid use has declined anyway with the advent of acid-suppressant medication.

Excess acid is also said to encourage an inflamed colon (colitis).

Note that too little stomach acid can also cause indigestion. While some people with gastritis or a peptic ulcer make too much acid, most don't, and some make too little. Indeed, low acid is a major cause of peptic ulcers and gastritis. This is because it encourages *Helicobacter pylori* bacteria to inflame the stomach-lining cells and hamper their production of protective bicarbonate-containing mucus. It also encourages stomach cancer. Around two in five of us are infected, though only one in ten infected people develop an ulcer.

§ the alteration of the surface of its head so it can adhere to an egg.
This is done by fertilization-promoting peptide, a substance produced
by the prostate and mixed with sperm on ejaculation.

Capacitation occurs in the cervix or womb but occurs only if the alkalinity is right. This happens just before ovulation, when cervical glands produce 'sperm-friendly' mucus that is suitably alkaline, abundant, clear, elastic and watery, and contains strands that are aligned to encourage sperm penetration.

Action: Eat an alkali-producing diet to encourage favourable alkalinity.

Inflammation

Inflammation is part of many disorders, and research suggests it is encouraged by acidosis. For example:

> One study found a high-protein, low-carbohydrate diet (which is known to be associated with acidosis) increases C-reactive protein – a reliable marker of inflammation.
>
> (*Angiology*, 2000)

Action: Eat an alkali-producing diet.

Kidney disease

Acidosis can both result from kidney disease and encourage it.

> A study of 1624 women in the US Nurses' Health Study found that a higher intake of protein – particularly non-dairy animal protein – encouraged greater decline in kidneys already slightly impaired.
>
> (*Annals of Internal Medicine*, 2003)

> A review from the Indiana University School of Medicine associates a high-protein intake with increased urine protein,

sodium and potassium, and faster progression of chronic kidney disease. Such disease is often symptom-free, so anyone contemplating a high-protein diet should first have a blood test for creatinine and a urine test for protein. There are no clear contra-indications if this shows the kidneys are healthy.

(*American Journal of Kidney Disease*, 2004)

Alkalinizing the diet may slow the progression of chronic kidney disease:

A study at the Royal London Hospital found that kidney disease progressed rapidly in only 9 percent of people treated with sodium bicarbonate, compared with 45 percent of others. Those who took sodium bicarbonate were also less likely to need dialysis.

(*Journal of the American Society of Nephrology*, July 2009)

Action: Eat an alkali-producing diet.

Kidney stones

Calcium oxalate stones (the commonest type) and uric-acid stones (for example, in people with gout) are more likely with acidosis.

An Italian study of 187 people with calcium-containing stones found their diet's acid-producing potential was the biggest risk factor. The researchers suggest such people should eat plenty of vegetables and fruit but relatively little animal protein.

(*Urology Research*, 2006)

Studies show stones are more likely with:

- Type-2 diabetes.

- Metabolic syndrome (see page 101).

- Obesity.

Each can be associated with acidosis.

Consuming table salt – which is acid-producing – encourages calcium oxalate and calcium phosphate stones.

Sodium bicarbonate can alkalinize urine, making it more able to rid the body of uric acid without forming stones. Alternative urine alkalinizers include potassium citrate.

Action: Eat an alkali-producing diet.

Consider taking ½ teaspoon of sodium bicarbonate in a glass of water four times a day for a week, followed by ¼ teaspoon four times a day for 2 weeks.

Mouth ulcers

Sodium bicarbonate can soothe aphthous ulcers and aid healing.

Action: Dissolve 1 teaspoon of sodium bicarbonate in a glass of water and swirl a mouthful around your mouth every 2–3 hours.

Muscle cramp

Acidosis can draw magnesium from the body to accompany acidic anions, such as lactate, in the urine, encouraging cramp.

Action: Rest as necessary to allow your blood to clear its acidic lactate.

Eat an alkali-producing diet.

Consider taking ½ teaspoon of sodium bicarbonate every 6 hours if you get repeated cramp.

Muscle wasting

Ageing increases acidosis and is also associated with muscle wasting. The chronic low-grade acidosis that is so common in Western societies is thought to encourage muscle wasting.

> Research at Tufts University, Boston, involving 384 over-65s, suggested a higher intake of foods rich in potassium, such as vegetables and fruit, helps prevent age-related muscle wasting.
>
> (*American Journal of Clinical Nutrition*, 2008)

Action: Eat an alkali-producing diet.

Muscle fatigue and aching

Weakness and rapid fatigue during intense exercise are traditionally explained as being caused by muscle cells producing acidic lactate ions. Certainly during intense exercise the pH of muscle cells can fall from 7 to 6.8. But research shows that what actually happens is:

> During intense exercise, muscle cells eventually have to produce energy without using oxygen, which releases hydrogen ions and lactate. Hydrogen ions encourage cellular and generalized acidosis. Lactate can also move into the blood.
>
> (*American Journal of Physiology – Regulatory, Integrative and Comparative Physiology*, 2004)

If muscles didn't produce lactate, acidosis and fatigue would occur faster and performance would be severely impaired. This is because lactate is a very useful fuel for muscles as it produces energy so fast. Indeed, some athletes take lactate in a fluid-replacement drink before, during or after exercise. During exercise, the muscle pain known as 'the burn' is associated with a build-up of hydrogen ions and signals that lactate is enabling the rapid production of energy.

Most exercise-associated muscle cramp results from acidosis over-exciting nerve receptors in muscles. 'Delayed-onset' aching the next day results from muscle damage and exercise-induced inflammation.

Taking sodium bicarbonate before intense exercise can buffer acidosis, enabling more prolonged exercise. This 'soda loading' can reduce muscle fatigue and enhance recovery. But the large amounts often recommended (about 0.3g per kg body-weight) can cause symptoms (see page 90–91) and shave only seconds off performance time. So it is controversial.

A research review noted that performance improved for 400–800m runners, 200m swimmers, cyclists, and boxers who took sodium bicarbonate before an event.

(*British Journal of Sports Medicine*, 2010)

Muscle fatigue and aching unrelated to exercise can result from a slow-onset immune reaction associated with a food sensitivity enabled by acidosis (see 'Food allergy', pages 104–5).

Action: Eat an alkali-producing diet.

Consider taking sodium bicarbonate, but only with supervision by a qualified coach or a doctor.

Nausea and vomiting

This can be caused by metabolic acidosis (see page 66) with a pH below 7.35.

It's also possible, though unproven, that chronic low-grade metabolic acidosis (see page 71) can cause it too.

Nausea and vomiting can also be symptoms of alkalosis (see pages 69 and 70).

Another cause is a slow-onset immune reaction associated with a food sensitivity enabled by acidosis (see 'Food allergy', pages 104–5).

Action: If you suspect acidosis, consider taking ½ teaspoon of sodium bicarbonate in a glass of water every 3 hours.

Eat an alkali-producing diet

Numbness and tingling

These can be symptoms of either respiratory or metabolic alkalosis.

Action: Consult your doctor if it continues and you don't know the cause.

If your symptoms are associated with rapid breathing (hyperventilation) triggered by anxiety or pain, consider seeing whether it helps to breathe in and out of a large paper bag to raise your blood's carbon-dioxide level. You can then try to keep the symptoms at bay by breathing more slowly.

Osteoporosis

Osteoporotic bone is light and fracture-prone. The risk factors include age; too much or too little exercise; smoking; too little bright outdoor light; a lack of dietary calcium, magnesium, zinc, vitamins C, D and K, plant hormones or fibre; too much 'diet cola' (because of its phosphoric acid); early menopause; anorexia; and various medications and illnesses (including gut and thyroid disorders – some of which can result from acidosis).

Studies also implicate inflammation, which can result from acidosis.

Acidosis also impairs bone health by decreasing the activity of bone-building cells (osteoblasts) but increasing the activity of bone-destroying cells (osteoclasts).

Research suggests that acidosis may draw calcium from the bones to partner acidic anions in the urine.

Finally, researchers believe chronic low-grade metabolic acidosis from an acid-producing diet can be a factor. In particular, they point to a lack of vegetables and fruit:

> This review of acidosis strongly suggests that diet-induced chronic low-grade metabolic acidosis has significant adverse effects that might be counterbalanced by an alkali-producing diet.
>
> *(British Journal of Nutrition, 2010)*

> A review from the University of Illinois suggests the acid-producing effects of dietary protein are minor compared with the alkalinizing effects of vegetables and fruits.
>
> *(American Journal of Clinical Nutrition, 2008)*

Vegetables and fruit contain many 'bone-friendly' nutrients and have an alkali-producing effect.

Several studies suggest an alkaline supplement could have a similarly helpful alkalinizing effect. For example:

A study at Tufts University, Massachusetts, of 171 people aged 50-plus, reports that taking a supplement of sodium or potassium bicarbonate for 3 months reduced calcium and bone-turnover markers in urine.

(*Journal of Clinical Endocrinology and Metabolism*, 2009)

Action: Eat an alkali-producing diet, in particular plenty of vegetables and fruit.

Overweight and obesity

Acidosis encourages resistance to the hormone insulin. Normally, insulin enables blood sugar to enter cells. But if cells are resistant, blood sugar rises and the pancreas produces extra insulin to convert surplus sugar into fat.

Many conditions are encouraged by, or associated with, both obesity and acidosis. For example, obesity and acidosis each encourage heart disease, high blood pressure, strokes, diabetes, metabolic syndrome, heartburn, gallstones, pancreatitis, osteoarthritis, gout, kidney stones, asthma, fatigue, depression, sleep apnoea ('stop-breathing' attacks during sleep), underactive thyroid, absent periods, infertility and certain cancers (though any influence from acidosis is only suggested as yet).

Since acidosis also encourages obesity, it is tempting to speculate that this is a linking factor.

A hypothesis from the University of Bochum in Germany explains how obesity is related to acidosis and the production of potentially damaging free radicals (reactive oxygen-containing ions). It also explains how the latter 'oxidative stress' could be the link between obesity and diseases commonly associated with it – such as high blood pressure, diabetes, heart disease and strokes.

(*Medical Hypotheses*, 2010)

It would also be worth investigating whether acidosis is responsible for other conditions encouraged by obesity – including age-related macular degeneration (an eye disease), Alzheimer's disease, deep vein thrombosis, pulmonary embolism, pre-eclampsia (a pregnancy condition), high blood fats, polycystic ovary syndrome and liver disease.

People who don't eat meat – and are therefore less likely to have chronic low-grade metabolic acidosis – are also less likely to be obese:

A study of 37,875 people concluded that meat-eaters are more likely to be obese.

(*International Journal of Obesity*, 2003)

Another fact is that most obese people are malnourished. Severe malnutrition decreases the bicarbonate content of pancreatic juice, encouraging acidosis.

If you want to lose weight, be aware that for the same calorie intake you can eat an amazingly larger amount of vegetables and fruit than of foods rich in fat, protein and carbohydrate. For example, you could swap one 250g/9oz fat- and sugar-free muffin for 900g/2lb pineapple, half a melon, 2 pears, 150g/5oz grapes, half a kiwi, half a papaya and 2 wholemeal rolls! Or 200g of cashew nuts for 8 baked jacket potatoes.

Avoid a high-protein, low-carbohydrate diet, as this encourages acidosis. An added bonus of an alkali-producing diet is that you can eat more yet still lose weight, because eating more vegetables and fruit can turn a fat-storing tendency into a fat-burning one.

Action: Eat an alkali-producing diet.

Pain

Damaging factors such as inflammation, injury, heat, cold and lack of oxygen can trigger pain receptors by releasing a variety of agents. These include hydrogen ions (protons) and adenosine triphosphate (from damaged cells), serotonin and prostaglandins (from mast cells) and cytokines and nerve growth factor (from white blood cells called macrophages). Hydrogen ions cause local acidosis. These various agents act on specific receptors and on ion channels in the endings of sensory receptors ('nociceptors'). These receptors then send nerve signals to the spinal cord and brain, eliciting pain.

Pain is felt when damaged tissue has a pH of 7 or below (depending on its site).

It's likely that 'whole-body' (as opposed to local) acidosis encourages pain, too. So anyone troubled with pain of any sort – including headaches, period pain, sciatica and tendinitis – might benefit from changing the way they eat.

Action: Eat an alkali-producing diet.

Poor circulation

Research strongly suggests that acidosis encourages the narrowing and stiffening of arteries known as atherosclerosis (see 'Heart disease', pages 107–9). Although the body compensates for the obstruction to normal circulation by developing high blood pressure, atherosclerosis is eventually likely to reduce the rate of the blood supply. This, in turn, can strain the normal working of all the body's cells. Some of the most obvious of the many possible symptoms are:

• Abnormal sensitivity to cold

• Impotence in men

- Lack of libido

- Paleness

- Poor memory

- Slow wound healing (especially on legs, ankles and feet).

Action: Eat an alkali-producing diet.

Premature ageing

Scientists have long searched for lifestyle factors that encourage a long life and discourage age-related conditions such as wrinkles, age spots, arthritis, heart disease, diabetes, cancer, osteoporosis, age-related macular degeneration, cataracts, poor memory and Alzheimer's.

Long-lived peoples include certain groups in Russia (the Georgians), Pakistan (the Hunzas), Ecuador, China, Tibet and Peru. One link is that they tend to live at high altitudes and drink mountain water rich in alkaline minerals such as calcium, which help prevent acidosis. Another is their consumption of fermented vegetables, fruit, milk, cereal grains, meat or fish. These contain acids (such as lactic, acetic and malic) produced during fermentation but metabolized to alkali in the body.

Another related fact is that spa water from medicinal springs is invariably alkaline.

In contrast, chronic low-grade metabolic acidosis is very common in peoples eating a typical Western diet. And ageing exaggerates acidosis because declining kidney function reduces the excretion of excess acid:

A research review found that ageing is accompanied by worsening low-grade metabolic acidosis, with an increase in blood pH and a decrease in its bicarbonate that may reflect the expected age-related decline of kidney function. Also, the blood's carbon dioxide concentration falls with age, because the lungs compensate for acidosis with more rapid breathing.

(*The Journals of Gerontology*, 1996)

The pH change accompanying acidosis has damaging effects on cells and metabolism in general (see page 61), some of which encourage premature ageing. For example, it is associated with structural changes in proteins, the oxidation of fats and a lower oxygen supply to cells.

Action: Eat an alkali-producing diet.

Restless legs

This may result from a slow-onset immune reaction associated with a food sensitivity enabled by acidosis (see 'Food allergy', pages 104 5). *Action*: Eat an alkali-producing diet.

Consider taking a dose of sodium bicarbonate (see page 88).

Skin problems

Theoretically, at least, acidosis can trigger or worsen various skin conditions. This is because it encourages:

- Itching

- Inflammation

- Allergy

- Infection

- Raised insulin (see 'Diabetes', pages 101–2), which encourages dry skin, and skin tags and dark skin on the neck, under the breasts and in the armpits and groin

- Pain from broken or inflamed skin.

One way of treating many skin conditions is to eat an alkali-producing diet to prevent acidosis.

Applying sodium bicarbonate directly to affected skin combats certain problems. For example:

> When 31 people with mild-to-moderate psoriasis took bicarbonate baths, almost all reported an improvement. The baths reduced itchiness and irritation so well that the volunteers continued their baths after the study.
>
> (*Journal of Dermatological Treatment*, 2005)

Action:

- **Allergic contact dermatitis**: reduce itching by applying a paste of sodium bicarbonate and water.

- **Cuts and grazes**: apply a paste of sodium bicarbonate and water.

- **Eczema**: have an alkaline bath (see page 92).

- **Fungal skin and nail infection (including athlete's foot)**: soak feet in a bowl of water containing a handful of sodium bicarbonate for 20 minutes daily.

  Or rub a paste of sodium bicarbonate and water into affected toenails or fingernails and leave it on for 20 minutes. Also, sprinkle sodium bicarbonate between the toes each day.

- **Heat rash**: apply a paste of sodium bicarbonate and water.

- **Insect bites and stings**: apply a paste of sodium bicarbonate and water. (Wasp stings respond to something acidic, such as vinegar; remember: B for Bicarbonate and Bee stings, V for 'Vasp' stings and Vinegar.)

- **Itching**: apply a paste of sodium bicarbonate and water, or have a bicarbonate bath.

- **Nappy (diaper) rash**: sit the baby in a bicarbonate bath for a few minutes then pat dry.

- **Small burns, or sunburn**: apply a paste of sodium bicarbonate and cold water to help prevent blistering and scarring. The cold paste takes heat from burnt skin; also, sodium bicarbonate dissolves endothermically (removing heat from its surroundings as it dissolves), which absorbs further heat.

- **Splits on the ends of the fingers**: rub in a little sodium bicarbonate powder if the split is moist or make it into a paste first with a little water if it is dry.

- **Splinter**: apply a paste of sodium bicarbonate and water, cover with a sticking plaster (adhesive bandage) and leave overnight to help draw out the splinter.

Stroke

Just as acidosis can encourage coronary heart disease and heart attacks (see pages 107–9), so too can it encourage arterial disease and strokes ('brain attacks' caused by blood clots or bleeds from cerebral arteries) in the brain.

An acid-producing diet is a possible contributory factor.

An analysis of 8 studies involving 257,551 people found a lower
risk of a stroke due to a clot or a bleed in those with a higher
vegetable and fruit intake. The results suggest that consuming
more than the recommended five helpings of fruit and
vegetables per day is likely to cause a major reduction in the
risk of a stroke.

(Lancet, 2006)

Action: Eat an alkali-producing diet.

Tooth decay and gum disease

Mouth bacteria encourage tooth decay because they feed on food debris
and produce acids that corrode tooth enamel.

Acidosis is another possible, though unproven, cause of tooth
decay. This encourages the kidneys to excrete acidic anions. The
alkaline minerals such as calcium that must accompany them have
to be drawn from bones, organs or even tooth enamel. Enamel thus
weakened decays more easily.

Bicarbonate inhibits the formation of plaque (a sticky layer of food
debris that can develop into tartar, which in turn encourages gum
disease) on teeth. It also neutralizes acids produced by bacteria, helps
prevent tooth decay, and increases calcium uptake by enamel.

Action: Clean teeth with bicarbonate-containing toothpaste or sodium
bicarbonate powder.

Tremor

This is a possible symptom of either respiratory or metabolic alkalosis.

Action: Consult your doctor if it continues and you don't know
the cause.

If your symptoms result from the rapid breathing (hyperventilation) associated with anxiety or pain, try breathing in and out of a large paper bag to raise your blood's carbon-dioxide level. If this helps, keep the symptoms at bay by breathing more slowly.

Underactive thyroid

Chronic low-grade metabolic acidosis may depress the thyroid gland:

> Swiss researchers found that chronic metabolic acidosis reduced thyroid function by decreasing the thyroid hormones triiodothyronine and thyroxine, while increasing thyroid-stimulating hormone. They suspect this might account for certain effects of metabolic acidosis.
>
> (*American Journal of Physiology*, 1997)

Action: Eat an alkali-producing diet.

A last word

It Is sometimes suggested, though hasn't yet been proved or disproved, that chronic low-grade metabolic acidosis also encourages:

- Hyperactivity in children

- Lupus

- Multiple sclerosis

- Myasthenia gravis

- Pre-menstrual syndrome

- Sarcoidosis

- Schizophrenia

- Scleroderma.

Useful addresses and websites

Ask a pharmacy (drugstore) to order bicarbonate of soda in amounts large enough for cleaning. Or order on-line from a source on the internet. Or use a source listed below.

UK

Arm & Hammer

www.armandhammer.co.uk – information about their various tooth-pastes that contain bicarbonate of soda (baking soda)

United States

Arm & Hammer

www.armandhammer.com – email via the website to find your nearest supplier, or buy the products at your nearest Walmart, Costco, Home Depot or Lowe's.

Supplies bicarbonate of soda (baking soda) and various laundry and personal- and pet-care products that contain this substance. For example, their 20oz FridgeFreezer Pack, which has non-spill vents on three sides of the box, so it won't spill when you leave it open to freshen your refrigerator.

Bob's Red Mill

www.bobsredmill.com – find your nearest supplier.
Supplies aluminium- and gluten-free baking powder in large
amounts (4½lb bags) for cooking. This could be useful for anyone
concerned about unproven suggestions that aluminium (aluminum)
encourages Alzheimer's disease, and for anyone who is sensitive to
the cereal protein gluten.

The Diet Plate

Visit www.thedietplate.com (UK), www.dietplate.us (US) or www.
thedietplate.com.au (Australia).

The Eatwell Plate

Visit www.food.gov.uk/multimedia/pdfs/publication/eatwellplate
0210.pdf for a downloadable image that will help you balance
your diet.

Index